LIANGONG

HEALING EXERCISES FOR BETTER HEALTH

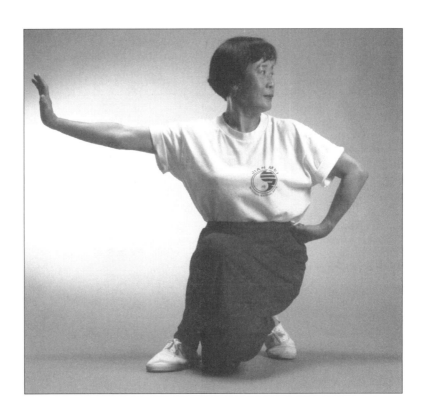

BY WEN-MEI YU

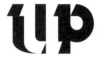

First published in 2003 by
CFW Enterprises, Inc.

Copyright © 2003 by
Unique Publications, Inc.

DISCLAIMER
Although both Unique Publications and the author(s) of this martial arts book have taken great care to ensure the authenticity of the information and techniques contained herein, we are not responsible, in whole or in part, for any injury which may occur to the reader or readers by reading and/or following the instructions in this publication. We also do not guarantee that the techniques and illustrations described in this book will be safe and effective in a self-defense or training situation. It is understood that there exists a potential for injury when using or demonstrating the techniques herein described. It is essential that before following any of the activities, physical or otherwise, herein described, the reader or readers first should consult his or her physician for advice on whether practicing or using the techniques described in this publication could cause injury, physical or otherwise. Since the physical activities described herein could be too sophisticated in nature for the reader or readers, it is essential a physician be consulted. Also, federal, state or local laws may prohibit the use or possession of weapons described herein. A thorough examination must be made of the federal, state and local laws before the reader or readers attempts to use these weapons in a self-defense situation or otherwise. Neither Unique Publications nor the author(s) of this martial arts book guarantees the legality or the appropriateness of the techniques or weapons herein contained.

All rights reserved. No part of this publication may be reproduced or utilized in any form or by any means, electronic or mechanical, including photocopying, recording, or by any information storage and retrieval system, without prior written permission from Unique Publications.

ISBN: 0-86568-199-6
Library of Congress Catalog Number: 2002014254

Distributed by:
Unique Publications
4201 Vanowen Place
Burbank, CA 91505
(800) 332-3330

First edition
05 04 03 02 01 00 99 98 97 1 3 5 7 9 10 8 6 4 2

Printed in the United States of America

Editor: Dave Cater
Design: George Foon
Cover Design: George Chen

TABLE OF CONTENTS

4	Acknowledgements
5	Dedication
6	About Dr. Zhuang Yuan Ming
8	Preface
12	Chapter 1: **History of Liangong**
15	Chapter 2: **What is Liangong?**
18	Chapter 3: **Benefits of Liangong**
21	Chapter 4: **Basic Meridians, Channels and Acupoints**
28	Chapter 5: **Basics of Liangong Practice**
	Chapter 6: **Movements of Liangong**
38	Section A: Neck and Shoulders
52	Section B: Back and Waist
70	Section C: Hips, Knees and Ankles
86	Section D: Limbs
102	Section E: Tendons and Connective Tissue
121	Section F: Internal
146	Chapter 7: **Testimonials**
159	About the Author

ACKNOWLEDGEMENTS

I would like to thank Dave Cater for editing this book, and for his continued support and encouragement in many aspects of my work. Special thanks also go to Debbie Leung, Janet Aalfs, Michelle Dwyer, Federico Di Bartolo, and Annabelle Nye for their many hours of assistance in making this book possible.

Liangong class at the 2000 National Women's Martial Arts special training seminar in West Virginia.

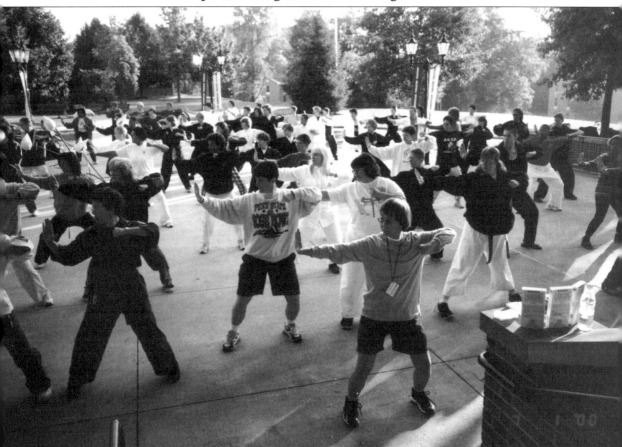

DEDICATION

This book is dedicated to my teacher and Liangong creator, Dr. Zhuang Yuan Ming. Without him we would not have Liangong; had he not taught it to me, I would not have it to pass on to others, who could then benefit from these wonderful exercises.

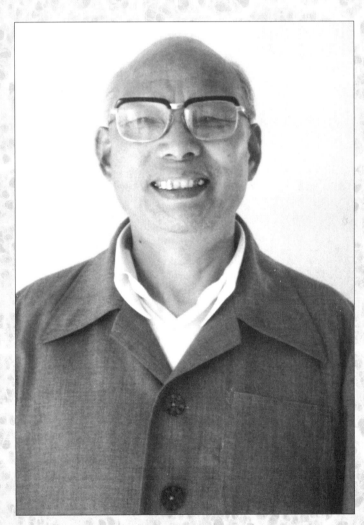

Dr. Zhuang Yuan Ming, creator of Liangong.

ABOUT DR. ZHUANG YUAN MING

Dr. Zhuang Yuan Ming is best known as the creator of Liangong in 18 forms. Born in Shanghai in 1919, he began his studies of traditional wushu at age 20 under the great Wang Zhi Ping. In 1945, under the direction and encouragement of his teacher, he began his studies of Traditional Chinese Medicine, specializing in traumatology (the study of the pathology and treatment of bodily injuries and hysteria).

Dr. Zhuang has devoted his life to improving the health of others. Liangong is the result of his studies and desire to create a system of exercises which has provided health benefits to millions around the world.

Wen-Mei Yu presenting a plaque to Dr. Zhuang at the 1992 Liangong Conference in Shanghai, China.

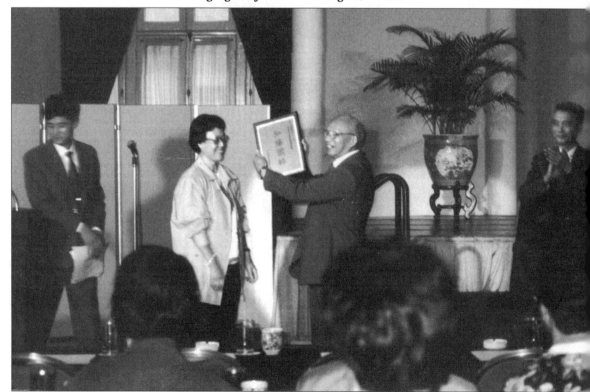

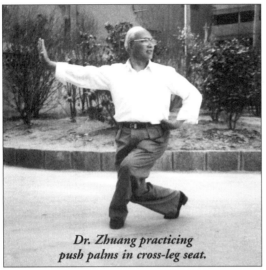
Dr. Zhuang practicing push palms in cross-leg seat.

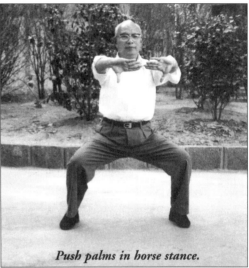
Push palms in horse stance.

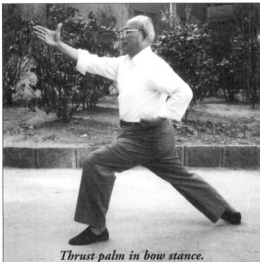
Thrust palm in bow stance.

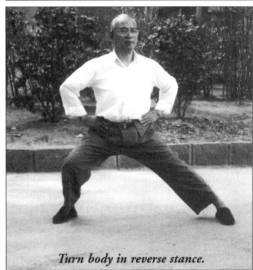
Turn body in reverse stance.

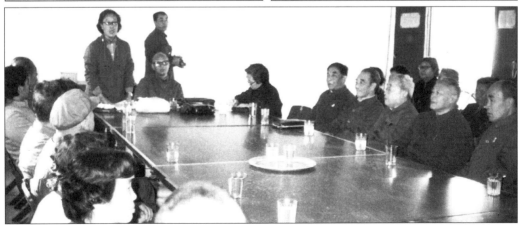
Special conference on Liangong attended by prominent masters and government officials, Shanghai, China in 1984. Wen-Mei Yu presents Dr. Zhuang, who is seated on her left.

PREFACE

Useful and easy to learn, Liangong is a modern health exercise developed from the ancient medical movement techniques of China's past. Its creator, Dr. Zhuang Yuan Ming, a doctor in Shanghai in the early 1970s, was familiar with both Asian and Western healing methods. He also studied martial arts under grandmaster Wang Zhi Peng.

Dr. Zhuang gathered a group of health professionals to help him refine Liangong early in its development. I lived in Shanghai then and joined this group as an established taiji and qigong instructor. My role was to teach the exercises, report my observations, and solicit student

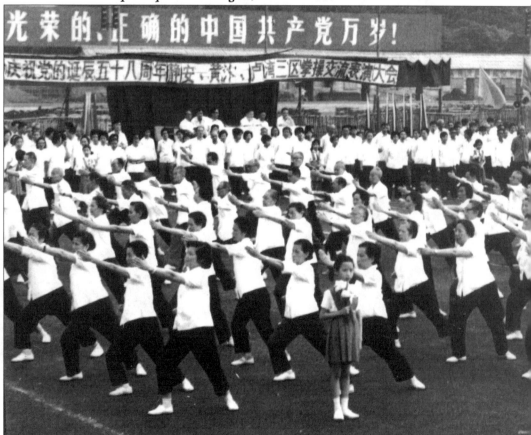

One thousand practitioners demonstrating Liangong in the People's Square in Shanghai, China in 1979.

opinions. Liangong was formally presented to the Chinese public in 1974. I continued to teach it as its popularity grew.

I moved to Southern California in 1987. A year later, I was injured in a car accident and experienced first hand the healing benefits of Liangong. I had pain in my neck and lower back, and a lawyer advised me to visit a chiropractor rather than treat myself solely with exercise and qigong, as I would have done in China. I got chiropractic treatments three times a week in the beginning; later I only went twice a week, but after six months there was still pain.

I then decided to try using Liangong to restore my health. It was

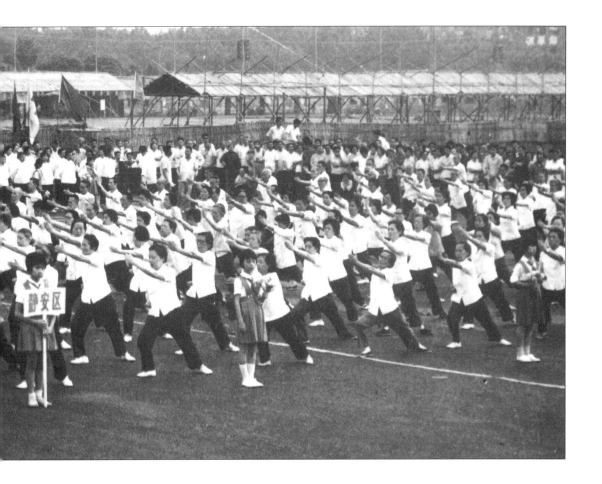

very painful at first but I continued to practice Liangong every day. After two weeks, the pain was gone. Experiencing the healing properties of Liangong strengthened my confidence and determination to teach it in the U.S.

People who desperately needed relief from pain came to me to learn Liangong. In the summer of 1992, I met Tina Chin, a real estate agent who suffered from nerve pain caused by a car accident. After seeing about 20 doctors over a two-year period, the pain continued to be debilitating. It woke her every night and any touch upon her body was painful. I taught her the first Liangong movements. In a couple of weeks, she felt better. A few months later, after learning more of the exercise, she was a new person.

Donna Honings, now a nationally known martial arts practitioner, approached me the following year. She wanted help recovering from a knee injury caused by years of incorrect kung-fu practice. After about three months of Liangong practice, her knee felt restored.

I began to see how Liangong could benefit many people in the U.S. So many experience pain and other ailments from stressful lives. Liangong can relieve pain acquired from repetitive movements, hours of sitting at computers or in offices, and awkward body positions, such as using a shoulder to hold a telephone against the ear. People can find relief from sports and work injuries caused by overuse, improper alignment and posture, and inadequate conditioning.

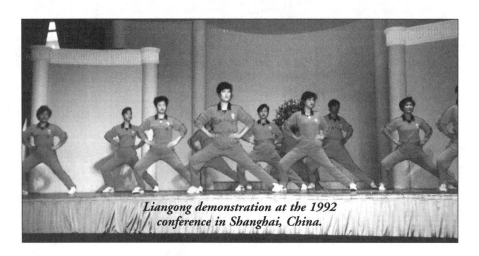
Liangong demonstration at the 1992 conference in Shanghai, China.

I want to share the benefits of Liangong with people everywhere. At workshops across the U.S. and Europe, students are enthusiastic about the benefits they feel almost immediately. Many later tell me about long-term improvements in their health and well-being after continuous practice.

The exercises are simple but the health benefits increase as more of its details, such as the alignment of the arms with the body and the straightness of the neck, are practiced with precision. To help people learn and remember the correct form, I produced instructional Liangong videotapes. Still, I received many requests for written information. With this book and the available videotapes, I hope more people will practice Liangong and experience its full benefits.

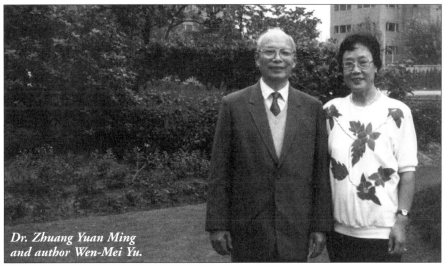

Dr. Zhuang Yuan Ming and author Wen-Mei Yu.

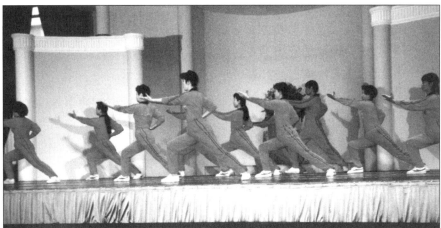

Chapter 1

HISTORY OF LIANGONG

Dr. Zhuang Yuan Ming, the creator of Liangong, is a chiropractor and tui na (Chinese massage and acupressure) doctor in Shanghai, China, who treats many patients daily. Chiropractic and tui na treatments usually provide some immediate relief from pain and symptoms of illness, but multiple treatments are often needed for a complete recovery and health maintenance.

Rather than relying on medical practitioners for continuing care, Dr. Zhuang contended that people could help themselves recover and remain healthy through exercise. He knew that ancient Chinese health exercises used movements to open channels and meridians for the proper qi flow needed to promote health.*

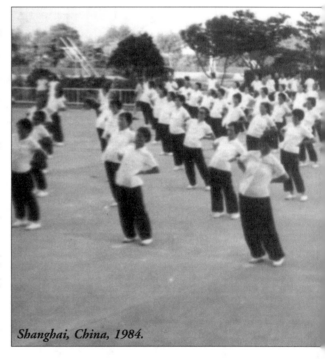

Shanghai, China, 1984.

Dr. Zhuang studied these therapeutic movement forms, the oldest created 2,000 years ago, taught to him by noted internal Chinese martial arts practitioner grandmaster Wang Zhi Ping. Grandmaster Wang had created an exercise composed of 20 movements, which he called 20 postures for prolonging life.

To create Liangong, Dr. Zhuang combined the ancient exercises of grandmaster Wang's 20 postures with his own clinical expertise, an understanding of the nature of common ailments, the curative methods of Chinese massage (tui na), and arranged the exercises in a more systematic way to work on specific areas of the body.

---

* Some of these old, often-esoteric sports therapies included Dao Yin (breathing exercise), Wuqinxi (five animals game), Baduanjin (eight section exercise), and Yinjinjing (muscle tendon change).

Master Wen-Mei Yu, an established taiji and qigong teacher, was recruited by Dr. Zhuang in 1974 to test the first 18 movements of Liangong, which became Series One. She taught these movements to the public, reported her observations, and sought feedback for Dr. Zhuang. She was part of an advisory group composed of doctors, professors in physiology and kinesiology, and other exercise instructors enlisted by Dr. Zhuang to help him refine the exercise. Dr. Zhuang also used this process to develop Series Two. Their work resulted in Liangong's current form.

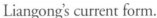

The first class had 50 students. More people joined the classes as word spread of Liangong's benefits. People liked the exercise and found its benefits easy to obtain. Relief from neck and shoulder pain was quickly noticeable. Liangong was easy to practice; it was not too lengthy and did not require much space.

Since 1975, Liangong has become very popular in China. Along with two other exercises, China's Ministry of Health, National Sports Committee and the All China Federation of Trade Unions selected it for popularization in 1980. One thousand coaching centers were established across the country.

In the 1980s, China encouraged skilled practitioners of its cultural arts to teach abroad and pass on an appreciation of Chinese culture to people around the world. Master Wen-Mei Yu, recognized as

China's excellent wushu coach in 1983, winner of traditional internal martial arts tournaments, and promoter of Chinese health therapies including Liangong, settled in suburban Los Angeles to share her knowledge and skills.

She impressed martial artists in the U.S. with her mastery of traditional taijiquan systems, revealed during demonstrations and victories at national and international competitions. Organizers of training seminars and workshops across the country hired master Yu to headline their programs. Practitioners in Europe soon heard about her knowledge and teaching ability. Wherever she taught, students of martial arts flocked to her to hone their taiji and qigong forms. In addition, everyone — martial artists of all skill levels, as well as the general public — found Liangong appealing and beneficial.

Liangong at Second World Tai Chi Day, Rose Bowl, Pasadena, Calif.

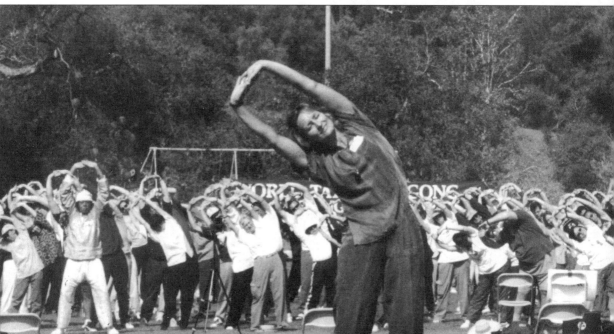

Chapter 2

WHAT IS LIANGONG?

Based on ancient Chinese movement therapies, Liangong, as a modern set of exercises, was developed to prevent and relieve health problems. It is divided into two parts: Series One and Series Two, each with three sections. The six exercises in each section focus on specific areas of the body, such as the neck and shoulders, or the joints. The exercises are generally simple and repeated on the left and right sides.

Series One systematically works down the body from head to toe as it strengthens, stretches, and increases the range of motion of specific areas. Section A is made up of six exercises that relieve pain in the neck and shoulders. The exercises in Section B focus on back problems. The hips and legs are strengthened in Section C.

Each section in Series Two works the whole body while focusing on joints, tendons, or internal organs. Problems with joints are remedied in Section D. Section E provides relief from pain in tendons and connective tissue. Section F features self-massage of acupressure points and certain areas of the body to prevent and heal internal disorders.

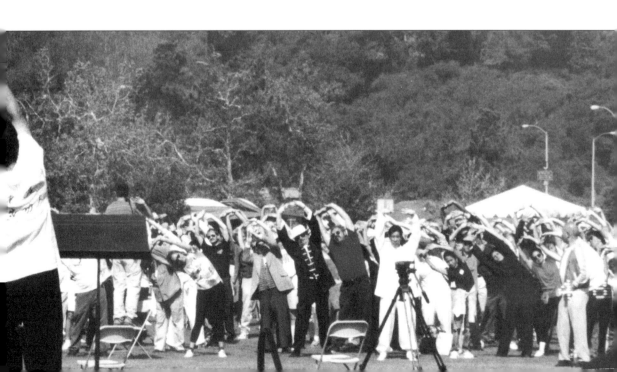

Although the time required to practice Liangong varies depending on the degree of individualization applied to meet particular health needs, it generally takes 20 minutes to do the entire set of exercises.

Very little space is required to practice Liangong. In many of its exercises, the feet remain stationary while the arms and body stretch in all directions. A few exercises require a wide step to the left or right, while one exercise asks the practitioner to take two walking steps forward.

HOW LIANGONG DIFFERS FROM QIGONG AND TAIJI

Liangong applies the methods used in qigong to strengthen qi flow and open the channels, meridians, and acupuncture points. But unlike qigong, Liangong uses a technique of tightening then relaxing the muscles in coordination with a holding and releasing of breath to push the qi through areas of stagnation. Along with a precise alignment of the body, this method produces specific sensations that indicate the production of internal energy. Practitioners usually feel health benefits quickly.

In contrast, most qigong forms stress relaxation to improve qi flow. Very few qigong sets have periods of muscle tightening and release.

The movements of taiji, a high level of qigong, are always relaxed and continuous and include martial applications that require a difficult coordination of the upper and lower body with the arms and legs. Perfecting the proper coordination of taiji's complex movements must be achieved before the relaxation required to attain the intended health benefits can be summoned. Taiji demands dedicated practice.

Unlike the continuous movements of taiji, Liangong is divided into separate exercises. They are simple movements focused on promoting the health of one part of the body. The exercises are completed one at a time, independent of the others.

Taiji and qigong forms promote health throughout the body.

When practiced in its entirety, Liangong's set of 36 exercises accomplishes the same purpose. But individual Liangong exercises, developed to prevent or heal problems in specific areas, can be singled out and used as a separate program to meets a person's particular needs.

Qigong systems have specific requirements regarding when they may be practiced. Practicing more than one qigong form within a 12- or 24-hour period can cause health problems because of the particular flow of qi produced by each form. In contrast, Liangong may be done at any time, even as a warm-up to performing qigong or taiji.

Liangong seminar in Toronto, Canada.

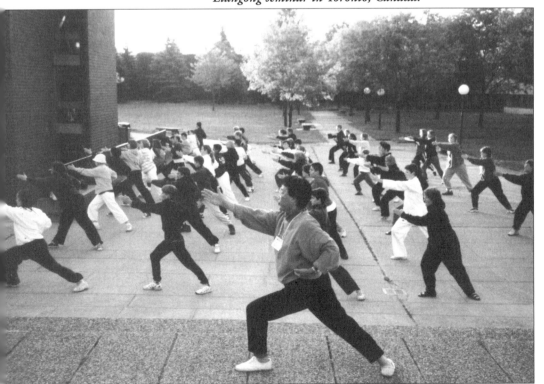

Chapter 3

BENEFITS OF LIANGONG

Liangong was created to prevent and relieve pain in the neck, shoulders, back, and legs. Repetitive strain, overuse, trauma, disease, stress, or a combination of these factors are often the cause of pain. Liangong prevents and reduces pain through gentle stretching controlled by the practitioner, increases range of motion, improves balance, increases muscular strength, and develops internal strength.

It develops internal strength by restoring and maintaining the proper flow of qi, generally defined by traditional Chinese medicine as fundamental life energy. People also claim success in the control of chronic illness after daily Liangong practice.

Where pain and health problems exist, Liangong can relieve and heal. For healthy people, it maintains vitality and prevents illness. The exercises may be practiced safely any time of day, as often as desired while monitoring excessive strain and fatigue, and in combination with other movement arts or therapies.

**LIANGONG'S FOUR APPROACHES
TO OBTAINING HEALTH BENEFITS:**
  1. **Each exercise in Liangong is designed for a specific purpose.**
  Liangong's six sections, each with six exercises, were developed to relieve pain in a particular area of the body by examining its anatomical and physiological characteristics. Unlike other Chinese therapeutic exercises that provide benefits to the body in general, Liangong practitioners can individualize their practice based on the location and severity of their health problems.

  Practicing Liangong in its entirety builds overall health and fitness while preventing pain and illness. When seeking relief from pain in specific areas, sections may be practiced alone or repeated while working the whole Liangong set.

In the three sections that comprise Series One, the first treats problems in the neck and shoulders. Back problems are addressed in the second section. The third section strengthens the hips and legs. Series Two begins with a section focusing on joints. Its middle section relieves pain in tendons and connective tissue, while the last section is designed to prevent and heal internal disorders.

2. Relieving health problems and maintaining health are achieved by developing internal energy.

Smoothly flowing qi is the basis for good health in traditional Chinese medical theory. Liangong works to strengthen qi flow along channels and meridians through precise body alignment, breath control, and the contraction and relaxation of muscles.

The traditional Chinese medical diagnosis for pain in the neck, shoulders, waist, and legs is usually "retardation of qi and stagnation of blood;" its symptoms include spasm, adhesions, and tightness in muscles, ligaments, and tendons. When practicing Liangong, qi is strengthened and pushed to the extremities, causing stagnant blood to circulate and generating internal energy.

Each Liangong exercise produces specific physical sensations when internal energy is generated. These sensations signal the proper execution of Liangong exercises for therapeutic results.

3. Combining Liangong with other traditional Chinese medical treatments enhances the health benefits of all therapies.

Liangong treats pain and illness through exercise, incorporating acupuncture, acupressure, and Chinese herbal therapy along with exercise into a complete treatment plan enhances recovery. Multiple types of treatments employ different methods to strengthen and store qi while expelling negative factors. This increases resistance to disease and injury, strengthens the body overall, improves the therapeutic effect of medical treatments, shortens treatment time, and prevents recurrence.

4. Liangong's most important feature as a health exercise is its ability to prevent future problems.

Respected physicians in ancient China not only examined and treated patients, they taught them exercises to practice at home to control the development of existing diseases and prevent the occurrence of future problems. They followed the old saying, "A veteran doctor treats before the diseases occurs, an inexperienced one treats after the diseases occurs." Dr. Zhuang Yuan Ming developed Liangong according to this medical principle.

Regulating and repairing overworked muscles, activating inactive muscles, maintaining normal function within the body by combining motion and rest, and improving balance and coordination prevents pain. By maintaining vitality, Liangong postpones the general decline and weakening of bodily processes caused by aging.

Master Yu teaching Liangong in Olympia, Wash.

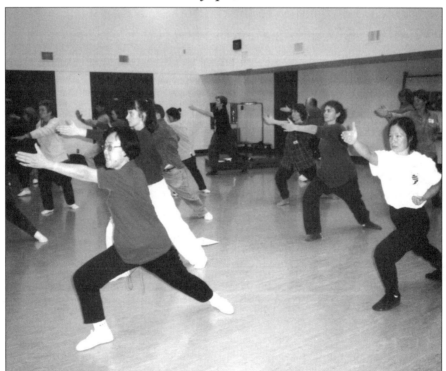

Chapter 4

BASIC MERIDIANS, CHANNELS & ACUPOINTS

Qi flows throughout the body within a special system of meridians and channels. It exists separately from the circulatory and nervous systems. The meridians and channels connect the body's exterior with the interior as well as its upper and lower portions. Points are sensitive areas on the channels and meridians that can be manipulated to affect qi flow.

The system of meridians and channels is like a road map. Similar to traffic in a city, qi is intended to flow smoothly. When a car breaks down or an accident occurs on a major thoroughfare, traffic is delayed or stopped altogether. This not only causes problems affecting the drivers in the traffic jam, but people throughout the city as well.

Similarly, a problem with the flow of qi can occur because of infection, injury, poor nutrition, and other problems associated with everyday living, such as pollution and physical, emotional, and mental stress. Qi is then said to be "stuck" at a particular location. Pain, stiffness, illness, depression, or other problems may arise.

The precise alignment of the body in Liangong's exercises corresponds to the flow of qi in the meridians and channels. When meridians and channels are aligned, qi can flow freely; if they are blocked, qi becomes stuck.

Knowledge of the most important aspects of the meridians, channels, and points will help Liangong practitioners understand the alignment required and the physical sensations felt when internal energy is generated. Opinions vary slightly throughout the world concerning the precise branches, locations, and paths of the channels, meridians, and points. Their locations can also vary somewhat from person to person.

ACU-MERIDIAN POINTS

Knowledge of a few basic acupuncture points will help in the practice of Liangong and serve as reference in describing the meridians. These points are the Baihui, Huiying, Laogong, Yongquan, and Mingmen. The precise locations of the points may vary among people just as physical features and bone structures differ.

• BAIHUI ("HUNDRED CONVERGENCES")

The Baihui point is at the top of the head, slightly behind the center. It can be found by moving the thumb and forefingers upward from the ears until they meet at the top of the head.

This point generally points upward to the sky, receiving Yang energy. Careful and correct stimulation of this point can relieve headaches, dizziness, sleeplessness, and high blood pressure.

• HUIYING ("YIN CONVERGENCE")

The Huiying point lies between the scrotum/vagina and the anus.

It usually faces down, toward the earth, thereby receiving Yin energy. Careful and correct stimulation of this point can help correct irregular monthly periods, provide relief from hemorrhoids, respiratory failure, and involuntary seminal emission.

• LAOGONG ("PALACE OF LABOR")

This point is in the center of the palm of both hands. When curling the fingers into the palm as when making a fist, it is where the middle finger contacts the space between the second and third metacarpal bones. The Laogong point also extends to the outside of both hands.

Because the hand easily moves to face up, down, right, left, front, or back, this point is used to emit and receive qi to and from any direction. Careful and correct stimulation of the Laogong point can help relieve cardiac pain and stroke complications, as well as stiffness of the tongue.

- **YONGQUAN ("GUSHING SPRING")**

Also known as "Pouring Spring" or sometimes "Bubbling Well," the Yongquan point is located in the center of the ball of the foot. It is the point of balance when standing with the heels lifted. Another method of locating this point is to draw a line between the second and third toe down the center of the sole to the heel. The point is one-third of the way down the foot from the top.

Like the Huiying point, the Yongquan point usually faces the earth, receiving Yin energy. Careful and correct stimulation of this point is good for correcting high blood pressure and relieving insomnia and headaches.

- **MINGMEN ("LIFE GATE")**

The vital Mingmen point is easily located on the lower back opposite the navel. In qigong practice it is essential to open this point to receive fresh qi, stimulate the channels, and strengthen vital organs.

The body's natural curve in the lower back closes the Mingmen point. Flattening that curve while relaxing the hips opens this point and can be achieved by lowering the center of gravity and gently tucking the buttocks while staying relaxed.

Careful and correct stimulation of this point can relieve impotence, involuntary seminal emission, and overcome menstrual disorders.

THE EIGHT MERIDIANS

The meridians are often seen as reservoirs. They have their own special routes but do not always follow a set sequential pattern as precisely as the 12 channels.

The meridians store any excess flow of qi from the channels, recirculating it in the channels as required. When qi is insufficient in the channels, the meridians deliver the qi needed to support the body's vital functions. The eight meridians help maintain the circulation of qi along the 12 channels.

Four of the eight meridians are important in understanding Liangong. They are: Du (Back Midline), Ren (Front Midline), Chong (Center of Body), and Dai (Waist).

• DU MERIDIAN (OR DUMAI; BACK MIDLINE)

Also known as the Governing Vessel, the Du Meridian travels along the midline of the back. It connects with the three Yang channels of the foot and hand as well as the Yang Wei Meridian. Because it is located primarily on the back of the body, which is considered Yang, it is known as the " Sea of All Yang Vessels."

The Du Meridian originates in the lower abdomen and comes out the perineum to curve around the anus, ascends the middle back through the Mingmen (Life Gate) point, and continues toward the neck. Continuing up the nape of the neck, it travels into the brain, passes over the top of the head at the Baihui point, continues over the head to the forehead, and down the column of the nose. It ends at the Yinjiao point located on the frenulum of the upper lip, the part that connects the upper lip to the gum.

Careful and correct stimulation of this meridian may help relieve rigid spine, shock, fever, coma, impotence, premature ejaculation, psychosis, and digestive diseases.

• REN MERIDIAN (OR RENMAI; FRONT MIDLINE)

Also known as the Conception Vessel, this meridian begins in the lower abdomen and emerges at the Huiying point between the scrotum/vagina and the anus. It then passes forward over the external genitalia, continues upward through the pubic region, ascending the midline of the front of the body through the abdomen, the navel, the center of the breast bone, to the throat, and to the lower jaw bone. There, it rounds the chin and ends at the Chengjiang point located below the bottom lip.

Careful and correct stimulation of this meridian may help relieve sterility, hernia, acute sore throat, urinary and genital diseases, profuse vomiting and diarrhea.

- **PULMONARY CIRCULATION**

Pulmonary Circulation is an orbit of energy achieved by connecting and circulating qi along the Du and Ren meridians. It is a smaller connection than the Systemic Circulation, which has qi flowing and circulating along all 12 channels.

The Du and Ren meridians are separated at the Yinjiao and Chengjiang points by the mouth. They are connected by letting the tongue gently touch the upper palate, which is just behind the Yinjiao point. Closing the lips and turning up their corners into a slight smile can easily achieve this.

One is cautioned not to concentrate too intently on this touching of the palate, or to use force with the tongue. Too much concentration or force can stop the qi, making the connection impossible and causing the pulmonary circulation to stop.

- **CHONG MERIDIAN
(OR CHONGMAI; CENTER OF BODY)**

The Chong Meridian, also known as the Flush Vessel, controls and regulates qi and blood inside the 12 channels. Some experts describe it as originating inside the body in the lower abdomen, emerging at the Huiying point, and ascending through the center of the spinal column. A superficial branch of the meridian passes up the abdomen along both sides of the midline of the front of the body, and then spreads through the chest, throat, and into the nasal cavity. This route is used for treatments along the Chong Meridian.

For qigong and Liangong, the Chong Meridian runs through the middle of the inside of the body, connecting the Baihui and Huiying points. When this meridian forms a straight line, qi flows up and down easily. Many Liangong exercises emphasize a straight, upright posture of the torso to activate this meridian.

Careful and correct stimulation of this meridian may help relieve sterility, uterine bleeding, abnormal rising of qi, spasm in the abdomen, coughing up blood, stuffiness in the chest, chest pain, and upper abdomen spasm accompanied by diarrhea.

- **DAI MERIDIAN (OR DAI MAI WAIST)**

The Dai Meridian, also known as the belt vessel, binds together all the channels of the body. The Dai Meridian originates just below the ribs and runs transversely around the waist. It activates, most often, when turning the waist during practice of Liangong exercises. Careful and correct stimulation of the meridian may help relieve abdominal tension, soreness and inability to turn the waist, numbness of the limbs and menstrual disorders.

THE 12 CHANNELS

The 12 channels are routes leading qi from the hands or feet to the internal organs of traditional Chinese medicine. Each channel has either a Yin or Yang character. One-half the channels are Yin, traveling through the interior of the body to Yin organs (solid organs). The Yang channels lie primarily on the outside of the body and lead to Yang organs (hollow organs).

The hand's three Yin channels lead to the lung, heart, and pericardium. Its three Yang channels lead to the large intestine, small intestine, and triple warmer (the three visceral cavities housing the internal organs). On the foot, the three Yin channels lead to the spleen, kidney, and liver, while its three Yang channels lead to the stomach, urinary bladder, and gall bladder.

Many Liangong exercises stretch the arms and legs, creating a strong sensation that runs from the tips of the fingers to the armpits and from the toes to the hips. These not only stretch the muscles, tendons, and ligaments, but also activate the channels, thereby strengthening the internal organs.

- **SYSTEMIC CIRCULATION**

When qi flows smoothly in all 12 channels, there is "Systemic Circulation." Achieving systemic circulation is not difficult. The channels will open and qi flow is stimulated when the natural forces of motion are coordinated with natural breathing. This is gentle breathing done in harmony with movement, in contrast to holding the breath in conjunction with isolated force.

- **THE THREE DANTIANS**

Qi is collected in three sensitive areas in the body called the Upper, Middle, and Lower Dantians. The Lower Dantian is where all qi is ultimately stored. It can be thought of as the "qi bank" where deposits and withdraws of energy are made.

The Upper Dantian is located in the head and generally centered between the eyebrows. The Middle Dantian is in the chest, centered between the nipples, in the middle of the breastbone. The Lower Dantian, located in the lower abdomen, is about three finger-widths below the navel.

Qi accumulated in the Lower Dantian wards off stress and disease, but the energy used to combat illness and deal with stress must be replaced. Continuous withdrawals without replacement will lead to a general shortage of vital energy that is needed to maintain health. Serious problems may develop when the shortage becomes acute.

Rest, good nutrition, and a healthy environment that leads to a contented life naturally replace and store qi in the body. Liangong and taiji are exercise therapies that strengthen the natural process and augment it when necessary.

Chapter 5

BASICS OF LIANGONG PRACTICE

• BASIC PALM POSTURES

LIANGONG PALM
Keep the four fingers together and extend the thumb.

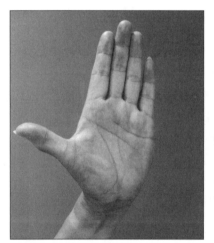

A. Erect Palm

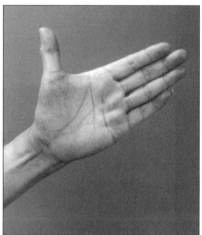

B. Thrust Palm

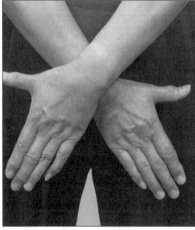

C. Cross Palms

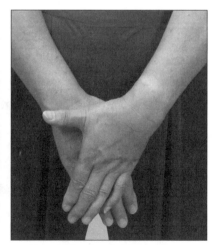

D. Stack Palms

FIST

Bend the four fingers and put the thumb on the index and middle fingers to make a fist.

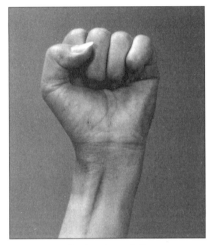

A. Surface of fist

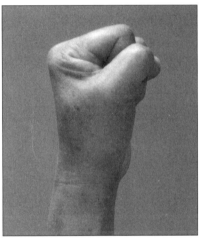

B. Side of fist

TIGER MOUTH

The curve made by the extended thumb and fingers in the Liangong Palm is known as a Tiger Mouth.

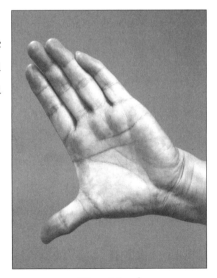

Tiger Mouth

• BASIC STANCES

UPRIGHT STANCE

Relax the whole body; stand with the body erect, feet together, arms at sides, eyes looking forward.

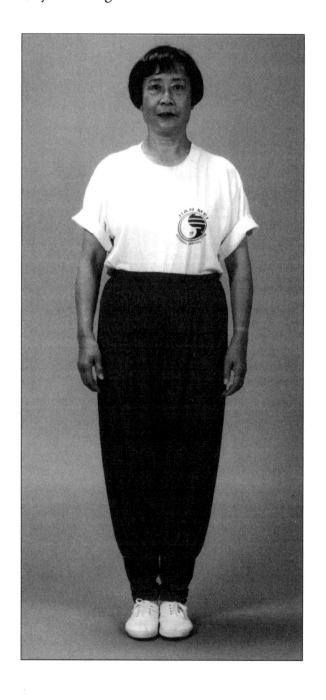

PARALLEL STANCE

Stand with the feet apart, parallel to each other.

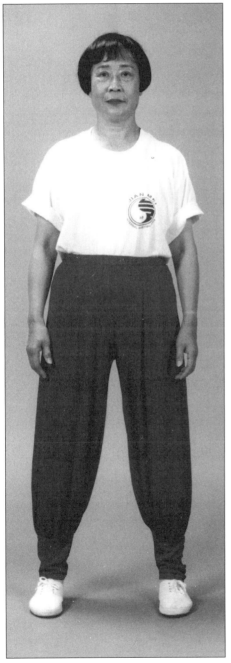

A. One shoulder-width apart

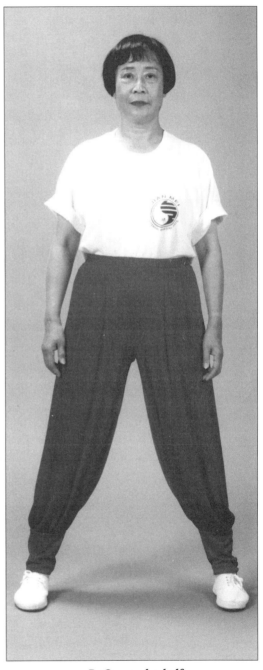

B. One-and-a-half shoulder-widths apart

PARALLEL STANCE

Stand with the feet apart, parallel to each other.

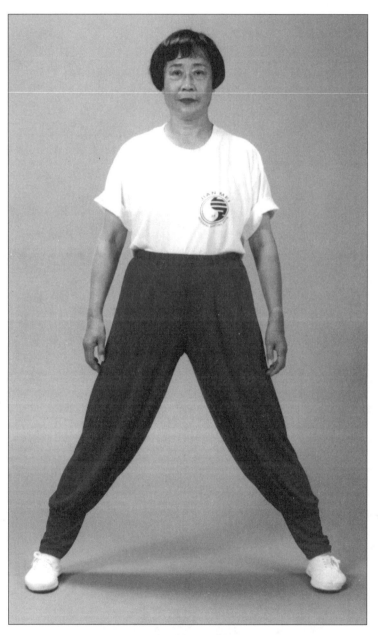

C. Two shoulder-widths apart

BOW STANCE

Parallel stance, two shoulder-widths apart. Turn one foot 90 degrees; bend the knee in line with the toe; straighten the other leg and keep the torso erect.

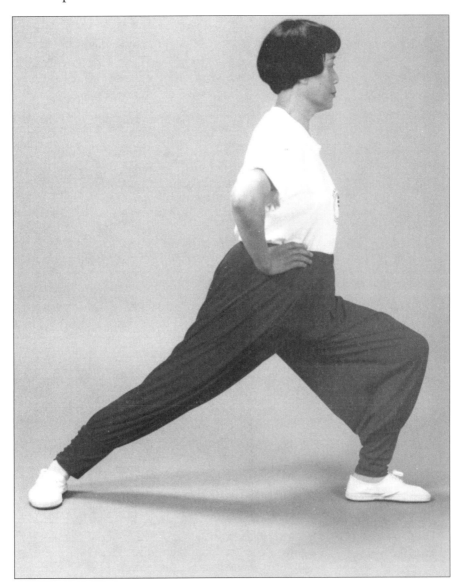

SIDE BOW STANCE

Parallel stance, two shoulder-widths apart. Bend one knee in line with the toe, straighten the other leg and keep the torso erect.

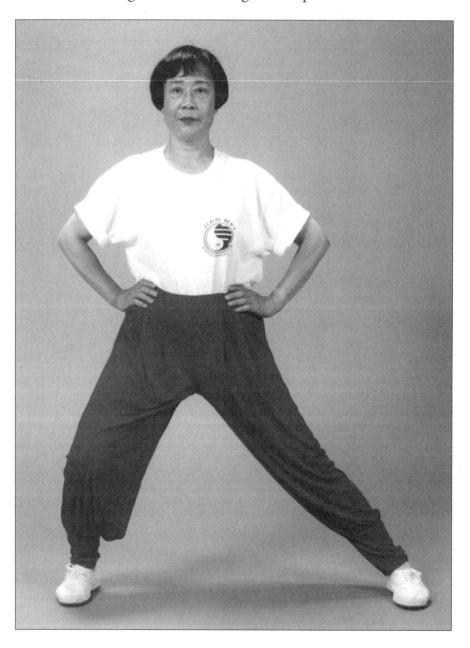

HORSE STANCE

Parallel stance, one-and-a-half shoulder-widths apart. Bend both knees in line with the toes and keep the torso erect.

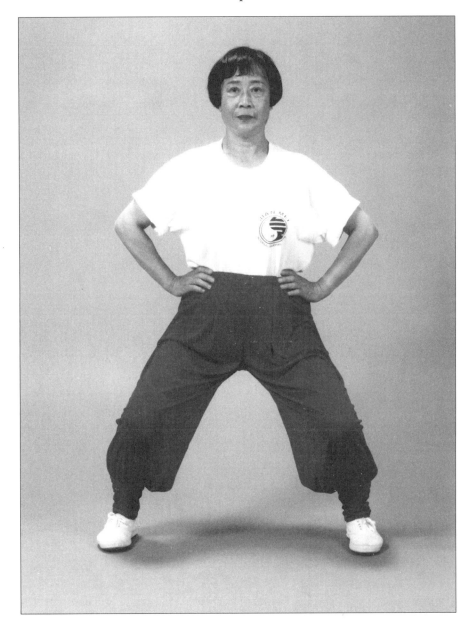

EMPTY STANCE

Weight on one foot, "empty" the other, keeping the torso erect. The "empty" foot: Only the heel or the ball of the foot is touching the ground.

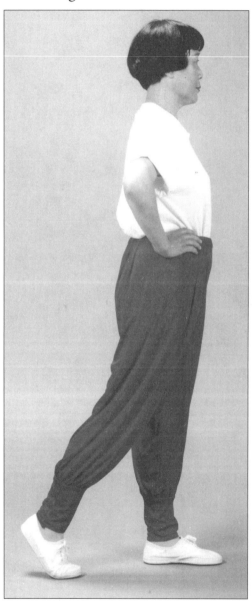

A. Weight on the front foot

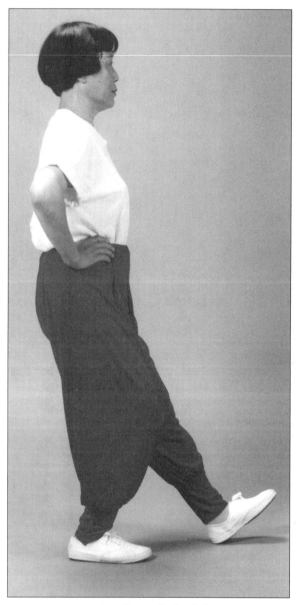

B. Weight on the back foot

CROSS-LEG SEAT STANCE

Cross both legs and squat down, keeping the torso erect.

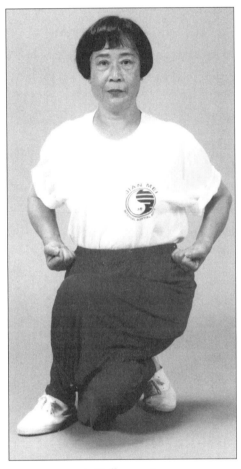

A. Full squatting

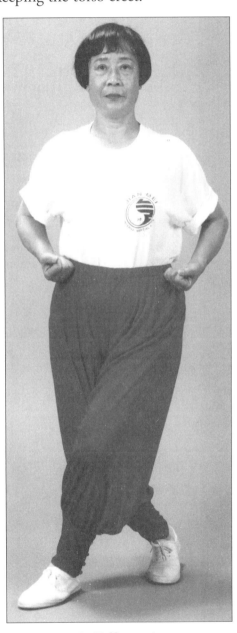

B. Half-squatting

Chapter 6

MOVEMENTS OF LIANGONG

TRADITIONAL THERAPEUTIC CHINESE HEALTH EXERCISE

SERIES 1

These 18 exercises prevent and heal pain in the neck and shoulders, waist and lower back, hips, knees and ankles. They help the body heal itself and improve strength and flexibility.

SECTION A
These six movements will help prevent and heal pain in the neck and shoulders.

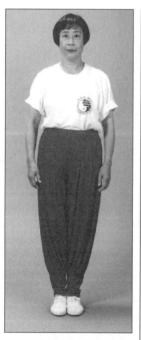

PREPARATORY POSITION
Relax the body, keep the body erect, feet together, arms at sides, and eyes looking forward.

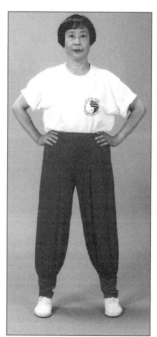

STARTING POSITION
The left foot steps out and is a shoulder-width apart. Parallel stance, hands on hips, thumbs pointing backward.

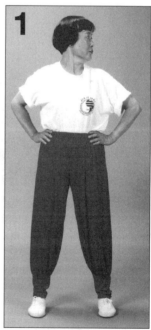

MOVEMENTS
Keeping the head upright, turn the neck to the left as far as possible.

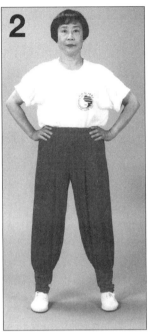
Return to the starting position.

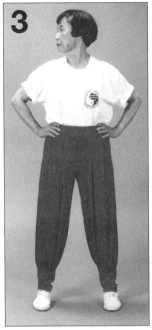
Keep the head upright, turn the head to the right as far as possible.

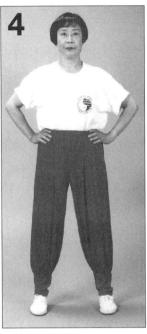
Return to the starting position.

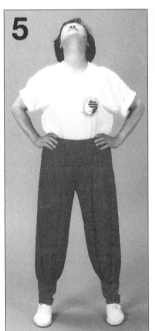
Lift the chin as far as possible and look upward.

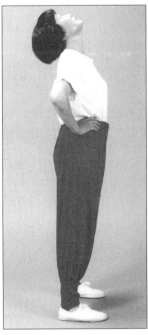
(Side view)

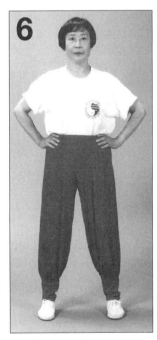
Return to the starting position.

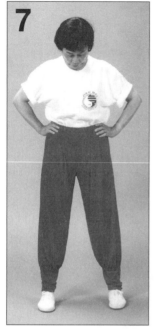 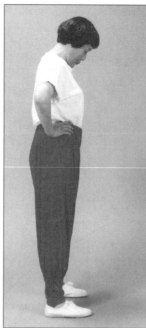 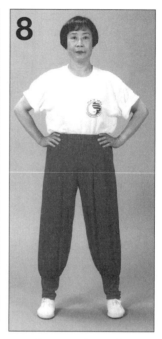

Bend the neck as far as possible and look downward.   *(Side view)*   *Return to the starting position.*

- **FREQUENCY**

  Do the eight steps two-to-four times.

- **MAIN POINTS TO REMEMBER**

  Keep the torso erect while turning the head left and right or up and down.

  Keep lifting the chin until the back of the head touches the top of the spine.

  Keep bending the neck until the chin touches the breastbone.

- **EXERCISE SENSATIONS**

  Tension in the neck muscles.

- **BENEFITS**

  Acute neck sprain (for instance, Lao Zhen).

  Chronic disease in neck tissue (as cervical syndrome).

  Relieves tension in the neck muscles and tendons.

DRAW A BOW ON BOTH SIDES

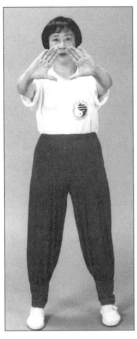

STARTING POSITION
Stand upright with the feet a shoulder-width apart. You are in a parallel stance. Palms are forward in front of the face about one-and-a-half feet away; "the tiger mouths" (hu kou) are facing each other and forming a round shape. (The hands form a small circle; the arms form a big circle.)

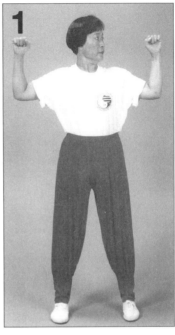

MOVEMENTS
Change the palms to fists at eye level; move out to align with the side of the body. The surfaces of the fists face upward. Keep the forearms straight up, the elbows pointing down; at the same time, turn the head left to look at the left fist, but focus beyond it.

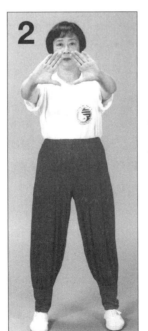

Change the fists to palms and return to the starting position.

DRAW A BOW ON BOTH SIDES *continued*

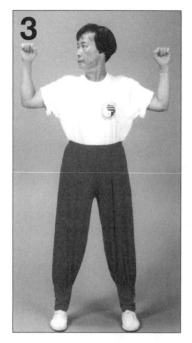

Same as steps 1 and 2, but in the opposite direction.

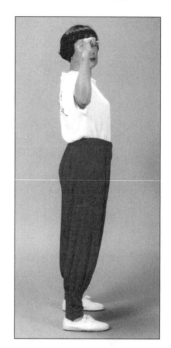

(Side view)

- **FREQUENCY**

  Repeat two-to-four times.

- **MAIN POINTS TO REMEMBER**

  Do not shrug the shoulders when separating the hands.

  Squeeze the shoulder blades toward the backbone and keep the elbows at the same level.

  Do not bend the wrists.

- **EXERCISE SENSATIONS**

  Tension in the muscles of the neck, shoulders and back while throwing the chest out and looking at the fist.

  Soreness can radiate to the muscle groups of the arms.

  There is a pleasant, soothing feeling in the chest.

- **BENEFITS**

  Relieves pain, stiffness and strain in the neck, shoulders, and back.

  Relieves numbness and paralysis in the arms.

  Relieves the stuffy feeling in the chest that accompanies colds, heartburn, and anxiety.

STRETCH ARMS

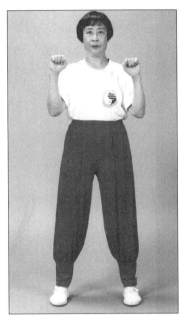

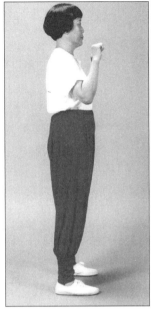

(Side view)

STARTING POSITION
Stand upright with the feet a shoulder-width apart. You are in a parallel stance. Bend elbows; both fists in front of shoulders, surface of fists facing upward, eyes looking forward.

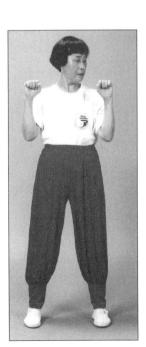
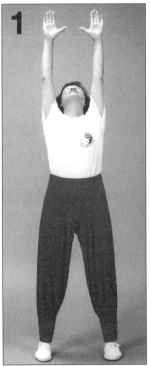
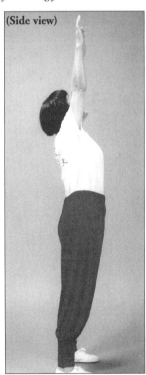

(Side view)

MOVEMENTS
1. Eyes look at the left fist; gradually change the fists to palms, raising the arms with palms facing forward, the thumbs facing each other, the fingers pointing upward, and the arms parallel. Lock the elbows. While stretching the arms, turn the head straight; look upward.

STRETCH ARMS *continued*

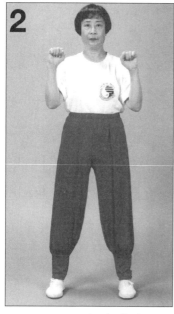
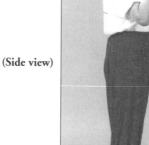

(Side view)

2. Gradually change the palms to fists; return to the starting position.

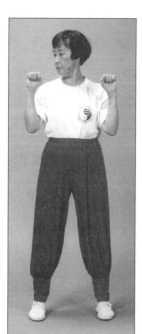
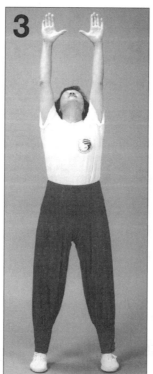
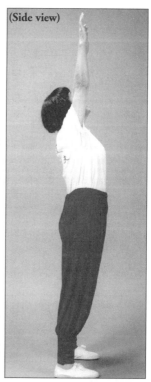

(Side view)

Same steps as 1 and 2, but in the opposite direction.

- **FREQUENCY**

    Repeat two-to-four times.

- **MAIN POINTS TO REMEMBER**

    While stretching the arms, thrust out the chest and pull in the abdomen; do not hold the breath too long. When raising the arms, keep arms, body and legs in a straight line.

- **EXERCISE SENSATIONS**

    Tension in the neck and shoulders when looking upward.

    Tension in the waist when thrusting out the chest and pulling in the abdomen.

- **BENEFITS**

    Relieves pain in the neck, shoulders, back and waist.

    Heals dysfunction of shoulder joints and stiffness in arms.

SPREAD CHEST

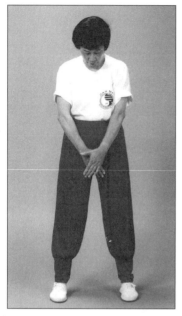
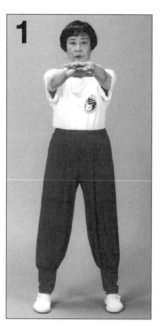
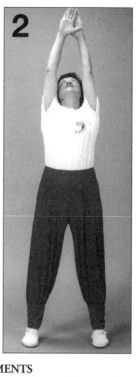

STARTING POSITION
Stand upright with the feet a shoulder-width apart. You are in a parallel stance. Stack the hands on top of each other in front of the abdomen with the left hand on top; look downward.

MOVEMENTS
Raise the stacked hands with the eyes following them (1-2).

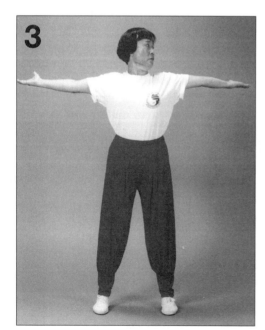
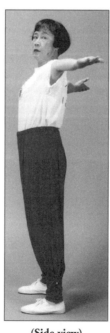
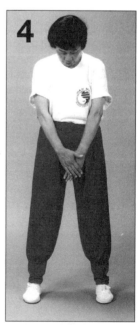

Separate the palms and circle the arms back behind the shoulders with the palms up; fully extend the arms, lock the elbows, and let the eyes follow the left hand to shoulder level (3).

(Side view)

Gradually rotate the arms, then return to the starting position (4).

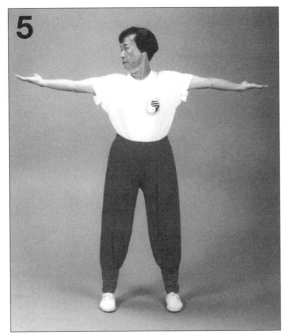
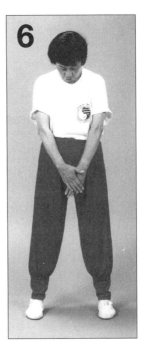

Same as steps (1-4), but in the opposite direction (5-6)

- **FREQUENCY**

  Repeat two-to-four times.

- **MAIN POINTS TO REMEMBER**

  While raising the arms, thrust out the chest and pull in the abdomen.

  When separating the palms, circle the arms back as much as possible.

  If you have pain in one shoulder, the hand on the top should be from the side that hurts.

- **EXERCISE SENSATIONS**

  Tension in the neck, shoulders, waist and lower back.

  While stretching the arms there is a pleasant, soothing feeling in the chest.

- **BENEFITS**

  Relieves pain in the neck, back, and waist.

  Relieves rigidity and functional disturbance of the shoulder joints.

SPREAD WINGS TO FLY

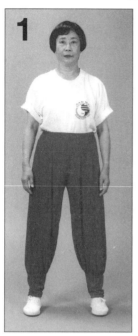

STARTING POSITION
Stand upright with the feet a shoulder-width apart (1). You are in a parallel stance.

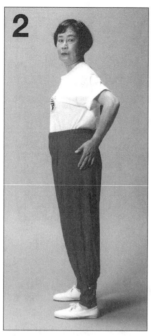

MOVEMENTS
Bend the elbows, draw them backward, turn the head to the left, and look at the elbow (2).

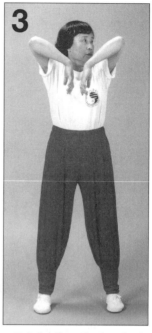

Lift the elbows by the side of the body like a bird spreading its wings for flight; circle them forward, keeping them at eye level; drop both hands in front of the chest (3).

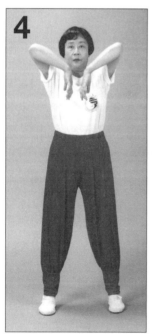

Turn the head and look forward (4).

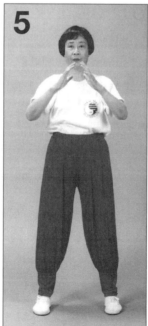

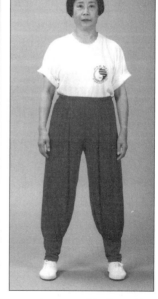

Slowly lower the elbows. The fingers point upward in front of the face and the palms face each other (5). Bring the palms down and return to the starting position (6).

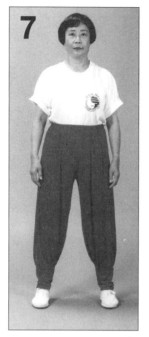 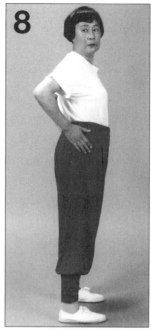

Same as steps (2-6), but in the opposite direction (7-8).

- **FREQUENCY**

  Repeat two-to-four times.

- **MAIN POINTS TO REMEMBER**

  Do not shrug the shoulders; keep the neck relaxed when raising the elbows.

  Do not stiffen or bend the wrists while practicing.

  Keep the head and body upright at all times.

- **EXERCISE SENSATIONS**

  Tension in the neck muscles, shoulders, and both sides of the chest.

- **BENEFITS**

  Relieves shoulder stiffness.

LIFT SINGLE IRON ARM

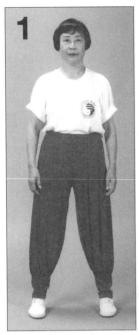

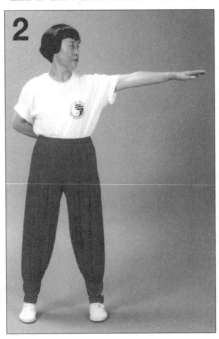

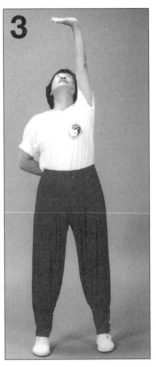

STARTING POSITION
Stand upright with the feet a shoulder-width apart (1). You are in a parallel stance.

MOVEMENTS
Turn the head to the left; lift the left arm sideways and upward over the head (2). Bend the wrist, palm facing upward, the fingers pointing 45 degrees back, and lock the left elbow.

Lift the chin; the eyes look at the back of the hand (3).

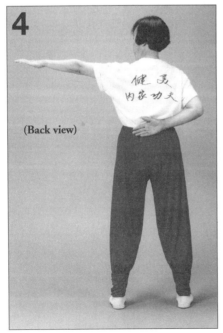

(Back view)

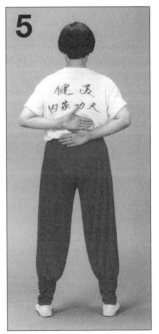

At the same time, bend the right elbow and place the back of the right hand on the lower back (4).

With the eyes following the left hand, lower the left arm sideways, gradually bending the left elbow and pressing the back of the left hand on the lower back above the right hand. Turn the head forward (5).

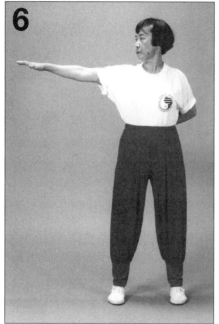 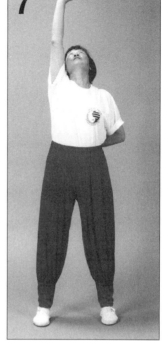

*Same as steps (2-5),
but in the opposite direction (6-7).*

- **FREQUENCY**

  Repeat two-to-four times.

- **MAIN POINTS TO REMEMBER**

  Do not move the body when turning the head.

  Keep the lifted arm straight, close to the ear, lined up with the trunk, and reach up to get a good stretch.

  The eyes follow the moving hand.

- **EXERCISE SENSATIONS**

  Tension in the neck and shoulders while stretching the arm.

  There is a pleasant, soothing feeling in the chest.

- **BENEFITS**

  Relieves rigidity and difficulty in moving the shoulder joints.

  Releases shoulder stiffness, pains in the neck, shoulders, back, and waist; improves digestion.

SECTION B
These six movements will help you prevent and heal pain in the back and waist (low back).

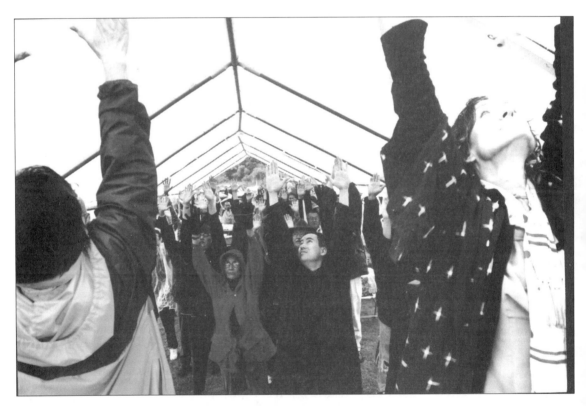

Liangong under pouring rain at the Third World Tai Chi Day at the Rose Bowl, Pasadena, Calif., 2001.

HOLD THE SKY WITH BOTH HANDS

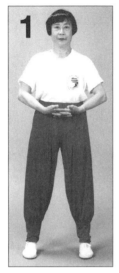
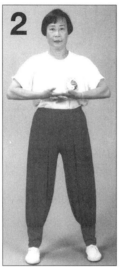
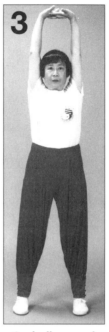
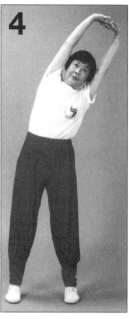

STARTING POSITION
Stand upright with the feet a shoulder-width apart. You are in a parallel stance. Clasp hands in front of the upper abdomen, palms facing upward (1).

MOVEMENTS
Raise the hands up to chest level (2).

Gradually rotate the palms up, reach above the head; lock the elbows, stretch the arms, and expand the chest (3).

Bend the upper body to the left (4) and return to an upright position (5).

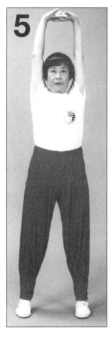
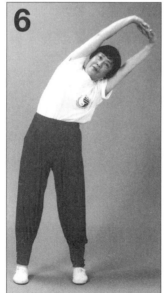
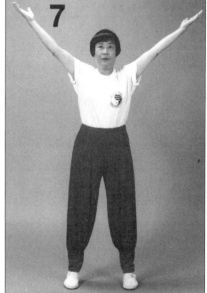

Bend the upper body to the left once more, but as far as possible (6).

MOVEMENTS

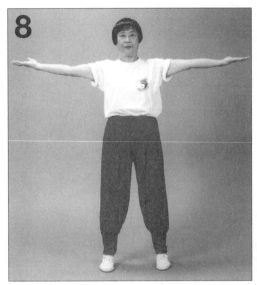
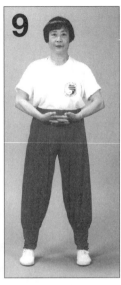
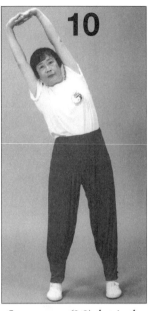

Lower the arms sideways and return to the starting position (7-9).

Same as steps (2-9), but in the opposite direction (10-14).

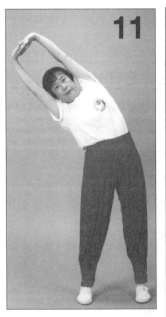
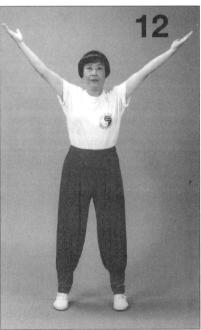
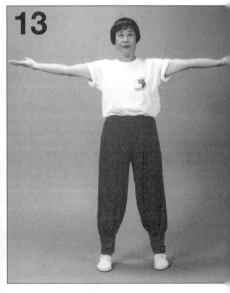

- **FREQUENCY**

  Repeat two-to-four times.

- **MAIN POINTS TO REMEMBER**

  Keep the arms upright and lock the elbows while the palms hold up the sky.

  When bending the upper body sideways, do not move the hips.

  Lock the knees when stretching.

- **EXERCISE SENSATIONS**

  Tension in the neck and waist, spreading to the shoulders, arms, and fingers.

- **BENEFITS**

  Eases stiffness of the neck and waist, relieves functional ailments in the shoulder, elbow joints and spinal column, and corrects a crooked spine. (Kyphosis, a backward curving of the spine, or a humpback.)

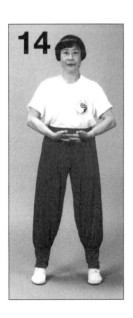

TURN WAIST AND PUSH PALMS

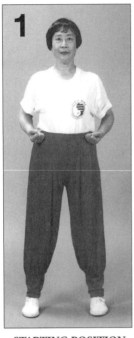
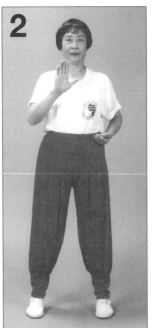
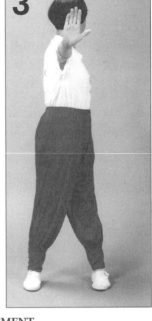

STARTING POSITION
Stand upright with the feet a shoulder-width apart. You are in a parallel stance, fists at waist level (1).

MOVEMENT
Open the right fist to an erect palm in front of the chest (2), and push it forward; at the same time, turn the upper body 90 degrees to the left without moving the feet. Turn the head to the left, with the eyes looking backward.

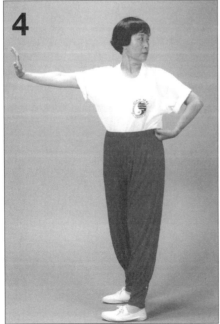
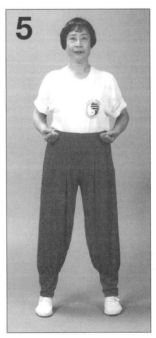

Bend the left elbow and place the surface of the left fist perpendicular to the waist to form a straight line with the right arm (3-4).

Gradually change the right palm to a fist and return to the starting position (5).

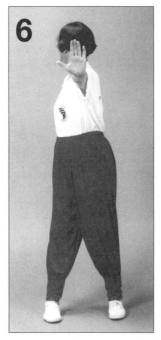 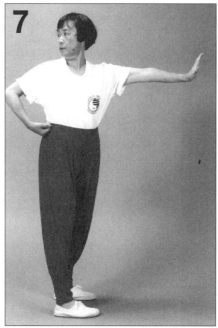

Same as steps (2-5), but in the opposite direction (6-7).

- **FREQUENCY**

  Repeat two-to-four times.

- **MAIN POINTS TO REMEMBER**

  Keep the body erect when turning the waist; do not move the feet; lock the knees and stretch both legs.

  Do not shift the center of gravity to the left or the right.

  When pushing the erect palm forward, try to keep the palm at 90 degrees to the arm; at the end of the movement, lock the elbow and stretch the arm. Do not shrug the shoulders.

- **EXERCISE SENSATION**

  Tension in the waist, shoulders, neck and back, also spreading to the arms and legs.

- **BENEFITS**

  Helps heal injuries of muscle tissues in the neck, shoulders, back and waist.

  Relieves numbness and muscular atrophy in the arms and hands.

CIRCLE HIPS

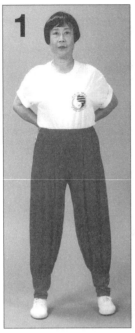
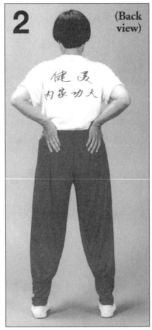
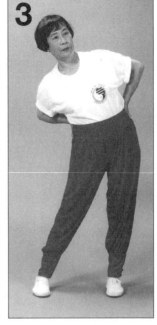

STARTING POSITION
Stand upright with the feet a shoulder-width apart. You are in a parallel stance. Place the palms at the waist, thumbs pointing forward, fingers pointing downward (1-2).

MOVEMENTS
Push the pelvis firmly to the left, rotating the hips in a complete clockwise circle (3-7).

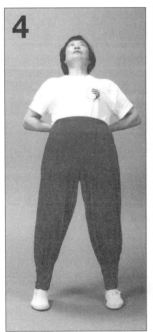
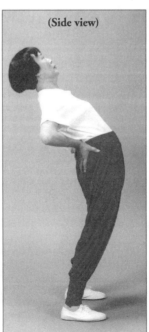
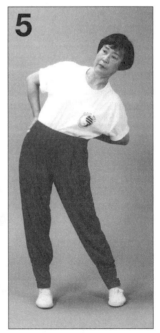

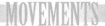

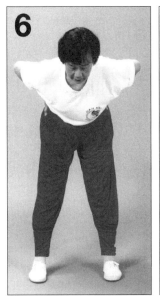 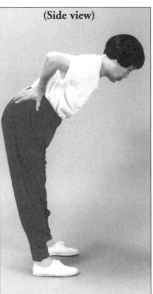

Continued on page 60

CIRCLE HIPS continued

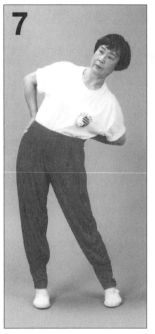 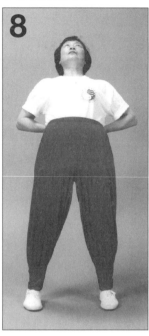

Same as steps (1-6) on previous pages. Push the pelvis firmly to the right, rotating the hips in a complete counterclockwise circle.

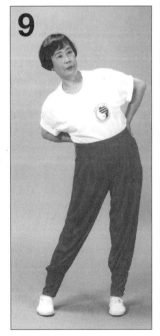 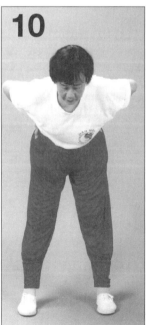 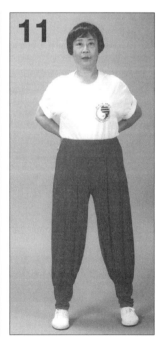

- **FREQUENCY**

    Repeat two-to-four times.

- **MAIN POINTS TO REMEMBER**

    Gradually increase the circumference of the rotation to the maximum.

    Keep the head in a straight line with the body while rotating the pelvis. Do not bend the neck at any time.

    Stretch both legs and keep the feet flat on the floor.

    When the pelvis is rotating forward, the upper body is leaning backward; push both palms forward into the back to help reduce the tension in the sacrospinal muscle.

- **EXERCISE SENSATIONS**

    Tension in the waist and lower back.

- **BENEFITS**

    Relieves chronic lower back pain and acute lumbar sprain; helps heal injuries in the lower back caused by occupations which require long hours of standing, lots of bending, and repetitive movements over long periods.

STRETCH ARMS AND BEND WAIST

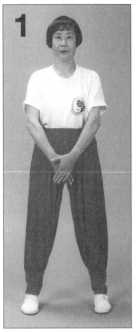
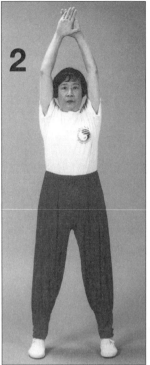
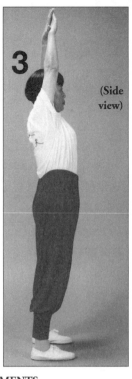

STARTING POSITION
Stand upright with the feet a shoulder-width apart. You are in a parallel stance. Put the left hand over the right in front of the lower abdomen, palms facing inward (1).

MOVEMENTS
Raise the hands forward and upward over the head, expand the chest and pull the abdomen in (2-3).

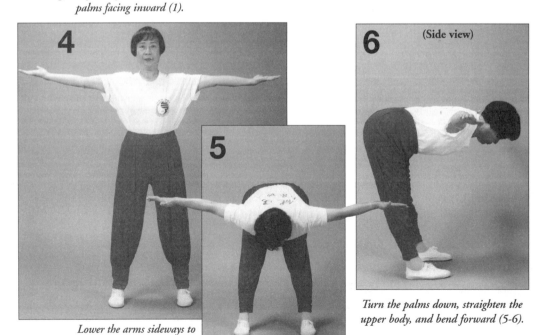

Lower the arms sideways to shoulder level, palms facing upward (4).

Turn the palms down, straighten the upper body, and bend forward (5-6).

MOVEMENTS

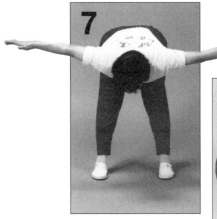

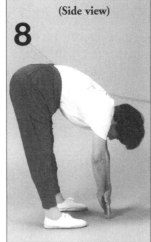

(Side view)

Stack the hands in front of the feet and try to touch the ground with the tips of the fingers (7-8).

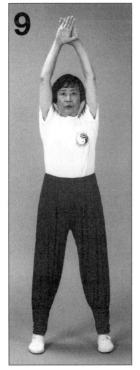

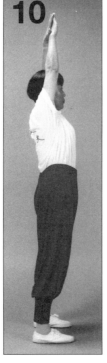

(Side view)

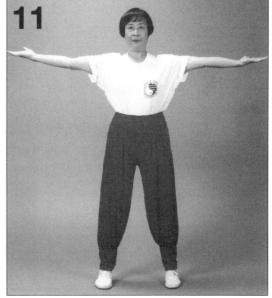

Raise both hands to head level, then straighten the body. Same as steps (1-2).

Repeat steps (5-8).

- **FREQUENCY**

    Repeat two-to-four times.

- **MAIN POINTS TO REMEMBER**

    Raise both hands in a line with the body.

    Lock the knees and stretch the legs when bending the upper body forward.

    While bending forward, thrust out the chest and pull in the low back (mingmen point area).

- **EXERCISE SENSATIONS**

    Tension in the waist and low back when raising the arms. Soreness in the posterior muscles of the legs while touching the ground with the fingers.

- **BENEFITS**

    Relieves pain in the neck, back and waist.

    Relieves shoulders stiffness.

- **SPECIAL ADVICE**

    Cardiovascular patients: do not bend forward too low; keep the head higher than the heart.

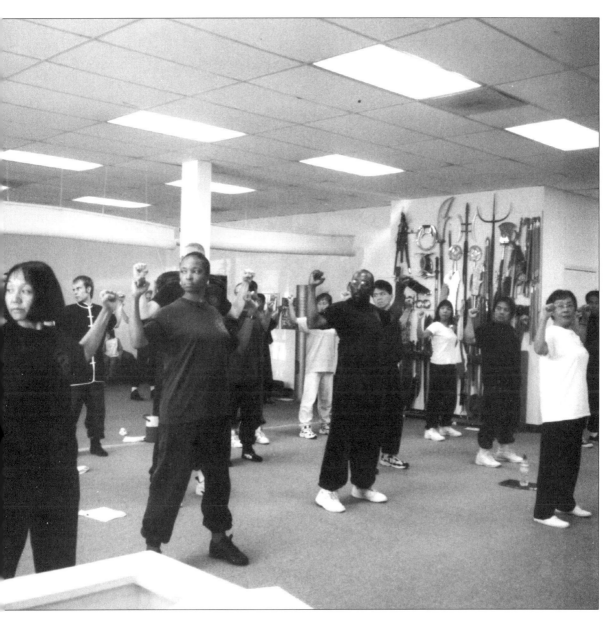

Master Wen-Mei Yu teaching Liangong at the White Lotus Kung-Fu Studio in Northridge, Calif.

THRUST PALM IN BOW STANCE

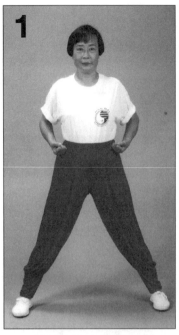

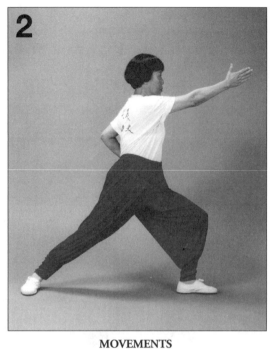

STARTING POSITION
Stand upright with the feet twice a shoulder-width apart. You are in a parallel stance. Fists are at waist level (1).

MOVEMENTS
Turn the upper body left, pivot on the left heel, turn the foot 90 degrees; bend the left knee and straighten the right leg (left bow stance). At the same time, open the right fist into a palm. Thrust it forward and slightly upward until the thumb tip is at head level (2-3).

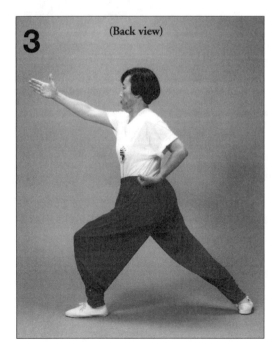
(Back view)

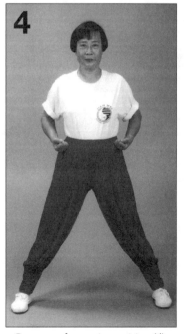

Return to the starting position (4).

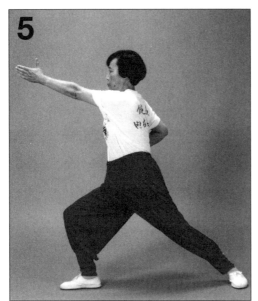
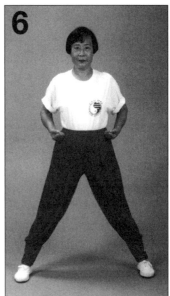

Same as steps 1-2, but in the opposite direction (5-6).

- **FREQUENCY**

  Repeat two-to-four times.

- **MAIN POINTS TO REMEMBER**

  Keep the feet wide enough apart in a bow stance, the bent knee in line with the toe; do not move the rear foot.

  When in the bow stance, keep the trunk erect; the extended arm and rear leg are straight.

- **EXERCISE SENSATION**

  Tension in the lower back, waist and legs.

- **BENEFITS**

  Relieves pain and numbness in the neck, lower back, waist and limbs.

PLACE PALMS ON FEET

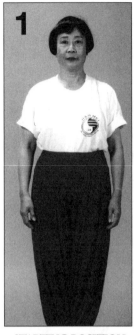
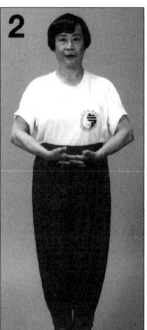

STARTING POSITION
Stand upright with feet together, arms at sides (1).

MOVEMENTS
Clasp the hands in front of the upper abdomen. The palms face upward. Raise the hands to chest level, gradually rotating the palms up and over the head; lock the elbows (2-4).

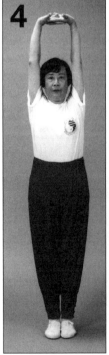
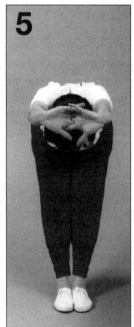
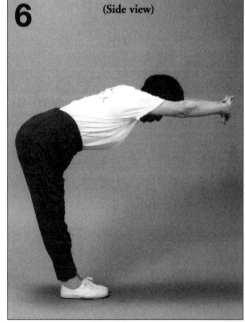

(Side view)

Gradually bend the upper body forward (5-6).

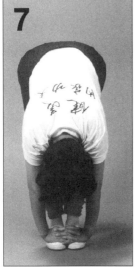 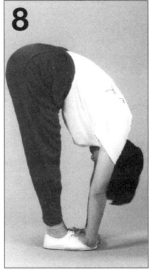 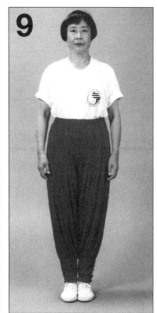

Continue to bend the upper body and lock the knees until both hands touch the feet (7-8).

Return to the starting position (9).

- **FREQUENCY**

  Repeat two-to-four times.

- **MAIN POINTS TO REMEMBER**

  Keep the arms straight; lock the elbows while the palms are up above the head.

  Do not lower both hands before bending the trunk.

  When bending the trunk forward and downward, thrust the chest out and pull in the low back (mingmen point). Move the buttocks slightly backward until both hands are touching the feet.

- **EXERCISE SENSATIONS**

  Tension in the neck and waist while stretching the arms.

  Tension in the lower back and legs while pressing the palms to the feet.

- **BENEFITS**

  Helps cure muscle tissue injuries in the lower back, waist and legs.

  Relieves stiffness of the lower back and waist and corrects a side-bent spine.

  Relieves pain and numbness in the legs.

- **SPECIAL ADVICE**

  Cardiovascular patients: do not bend forward too low; keep the head higher than the heart.

MOVEMENTS

SECTION C
These six movements will help in the prevention and healing of injuries to the hips, knees and ankles.

TURN KNEES

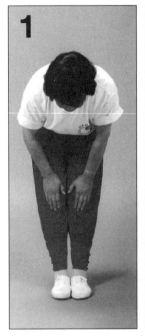
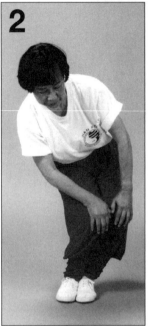

STARTING POSITION
Bend the upper body forward with palms on knees, feet together, eyes looking forward and downward (1).

MOVEMENTS
Bend knees to the left and start circling them clockwise (2-4).

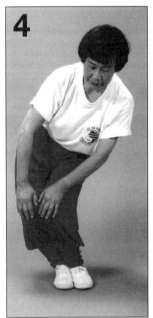
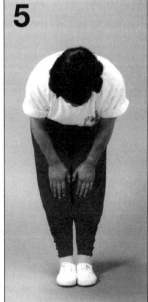
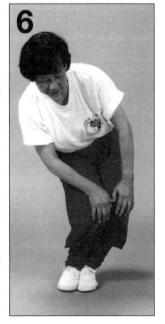

Return to the starting position (5).

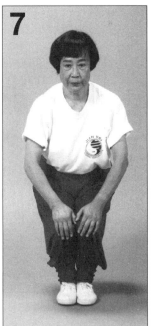 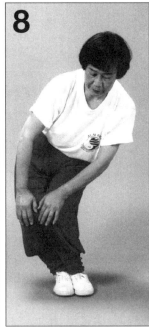 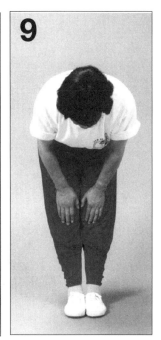

Repeat in the opposite direction; circle knees counterclockwise.

- **FREQUENCY**

  Repeat two-to-four times.

- **MAIN POINTS TO REMEMBER**

  Keep rotating at a steady pace. Move smoothly.

  Do not raise the heels during the exercise.

  When circling with the knees, the circles must be as large as possible.

- **EXERCISE SENSATIONS**

  Tension in knees and ankles.

- **BENEFITS**

  Relieves pain in the knee and ankle joints.

  Prevents weakness in the knees and ankles.

TURN BODY IN REVERSE STANCE

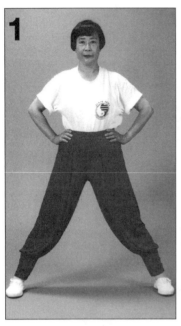
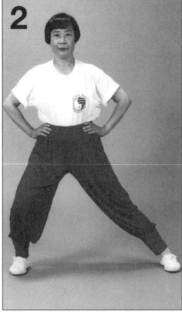
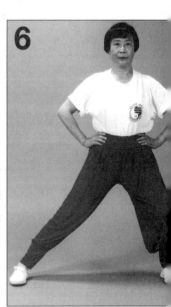

STARTING POSITION
Stand upright with the feet twice a shoulder-width apart. You are in a parallel stance. Hands on hips, thumbs pointing backward (1).

MOVEMENTS
Bend the right knee, shifting weight to the right leg, and then turn the body 45 degrees to the left (2-4).

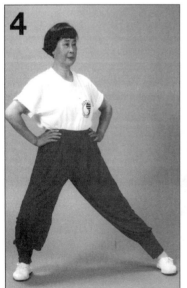
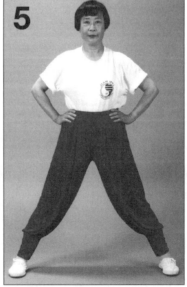
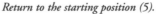

Return to the starting position (5).

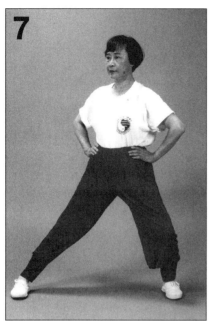

Repeat in the opposite direction (6-7).

- **FREQUENCY**

Repeat two-to-four times.

- **MAIN POINTS TO REMEMBER**

Keep the feet wide enough apart in a reverse stance; when the body is turned 45 degrees, keep the knee in line with the toe and the feet flat on the floor.

When one leg has the bent knee in a reverse stance, keep the other leg straight.

Do not lean forward, backward, or to the side.

- **EXERCISE SENSATIONS**

Tension in the medial side of the thigh (adductor muscles) of the stretched leg.

Tension in the femoral quadriceps of the bent leg.

- **BENEFITS**

Relieves pain in the low back, waist, hips and legs.

Helps with difficulty in movement in the joints of the hips, knees and ankles.

Helps atrophy of the muscles of the lower extremities; reduces difficulty in walking.

BEND, SQUAT AND STRETCH LEGS

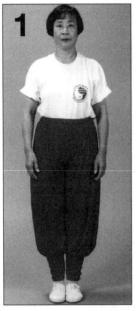
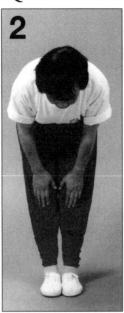
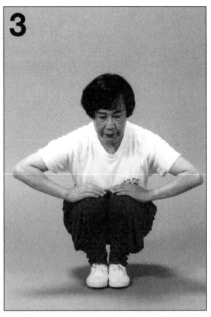

STARTING POSITION
Stand upright with feet together, arms at sides (1).

MOVEMENTS
Bend the upper body forward, placing the palms on the knees. Keep the legs straight (2).

Bend the knees and squat completely; at the same time, the hands are holding the knees with the fingertips pointing at one another (3-4).

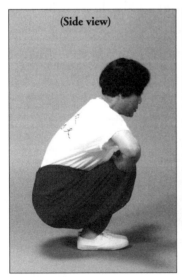
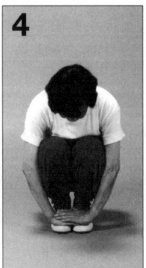
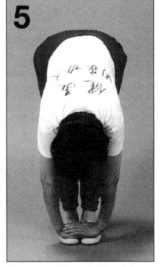

Place the palms on the feet, left on top of the right, then straighten the legs until the knees are locked (5-7).

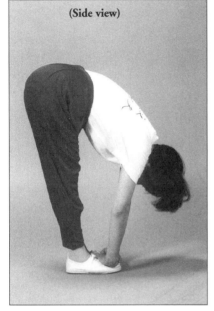 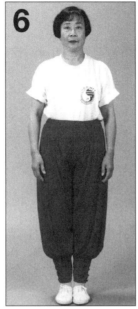 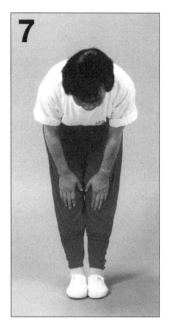

Return to the starting position.

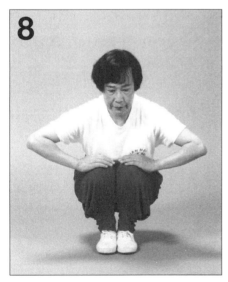 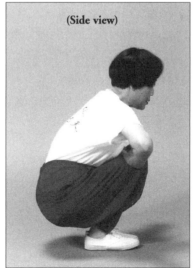

Repeat steps (4-5), but this time with the right hand on top of the left. Then return to the starting position.

- **FREQUENCY**

  Repeat two-to-four times.

- **MAIN POINTS TO REMEMBER**

  Keep the trunk upright when squatting fully.

  Use the hands to push the knees together to help the squatting.

  Do not lift the heels while squatting.

  When the knees are locked, press the palms as close to the feet as possible. After practicing for a while, you will be able to touch the feet when you straighten the knee.

- **EXERCISE SENSATION**

  Tension of the muscles of the front part of the thigh, and the knee joints while squatting.

  Tension in the muscles in the back of the thigh and calf while straightening the legs. Tension in the posterior muscle group of the legs when pressing the palms on the feet.

- **BENEFITS**

  Relieves stiffness in the lower back, waist and knees.

  Helps muscular atrophy of the lower limbs caused by difficulties in moving the hip and the knee joints.

  Relieves the pain in the flexion and extension of the lower extremities, sciatica.

- **SPECIAL ADVICE**

  Cardiovascular patients: keep the head higher than the heart when stretching the legs.

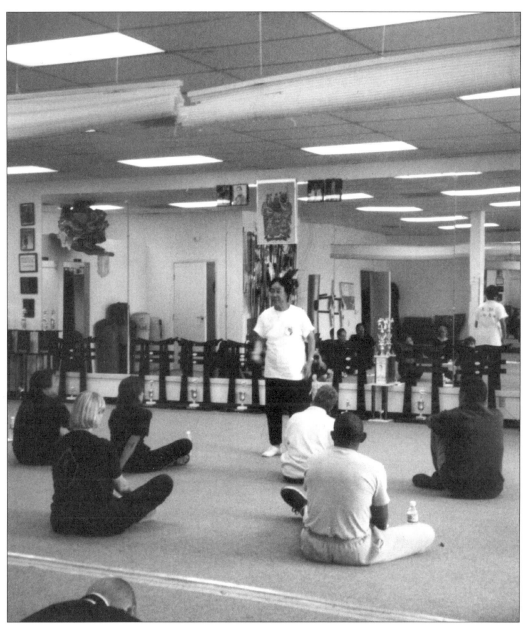

Master Wen-Mei Yu gives a Liangong lecture at the White Lotus Kung-Fu Studio in Northridge, Calif.

KEEP ONE PALM ON KNEE AND HOLD THE OTHER

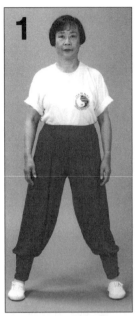

STARTING POSITION
Stand upright with the feet one and a half shoulder-widths apart. You assume a parallel stance with the arms at your sides (1).

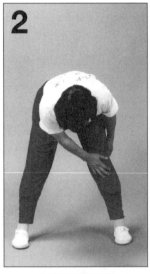

MOVEMENTS
Bend the upper body forward, placing the right hand on the left knee (2).

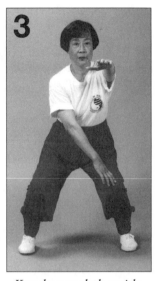

Keep the upper body straight. Lift the left arm from the front of the body (3) over the head. The palm is facing the upward, the fingertips pointing backward. Look at the back of the hand; at the same time, bend the knees into a horse stance (4).

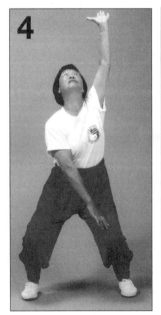

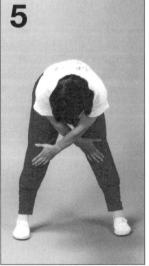

Bend the upper body forward; straighten the legs while the left arm crosses over the right arm. Place the left hand on the right knee (5).

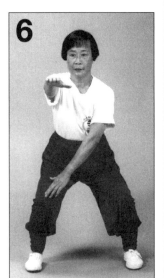
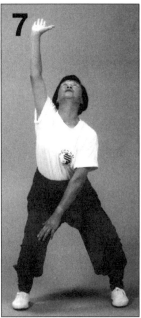

Keep the upper body straight. Lift the right arm from the front of the body over the head. The palm is facing upward and the fingertips are pointing backward. Look at the back of the hand; at the same time, bend the knees into a horse stance (6-7).

- **FREQUENCY**

  Repeat two-to-four times.

- **MAIN POINTS TO REMEMBER**

  Do not turn the waist when bending forward.

  Do not throw the buttocks out while bending the knees into a horse stance.

  Keep the upper body as straight as possible; do not lean to one side.

- **EXERCISE SENSATIONS**

  Tension in the neck, shoulders, lower back, waist and legs when looking at the back of the hand.

- **BENEFITS**

  Relieves pain and stiffness in the neck, shoulders, lower back, waist and legs.

HOLD KNEE TO CHEST

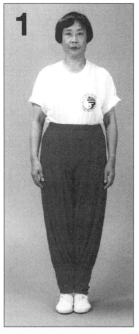
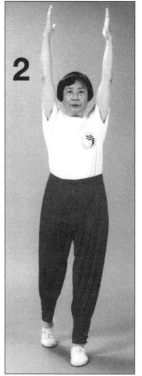
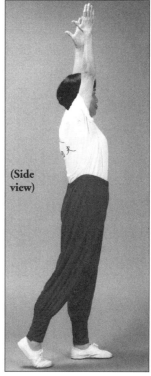

(Side view)

STARTING POSITION
Stand upright with feet together, arms at sides (1).

MOVEMENTS
Take a step forward with the left foot. Shift your weight onto the left leg and raise the right heel. At the same time, raise the arms forward and upward over the head with the palms facing each other (2).

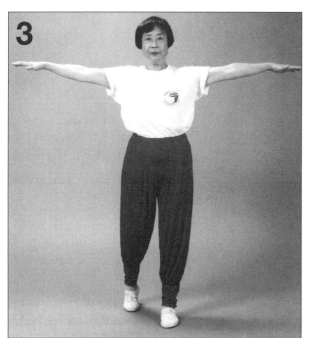
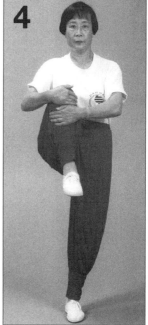

Drop the arms to the sides of the body (3); at the same time, lift the right knee and hold it up in front of the chest with both hands (4).

MOVEMENTS

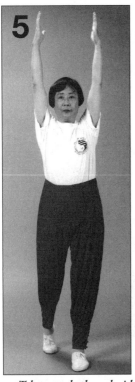
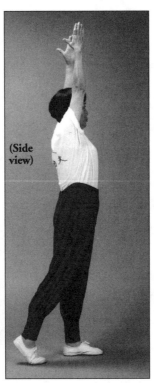
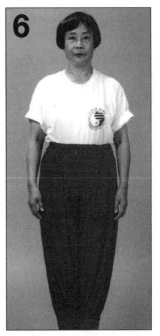

(Side view)

Take a step backward with the right foot without shifting weight. At the same time, raise the arms forward and upward over the head with the palms facing each other (5).

Take a step backward with the left foot and return to the starting position (6).

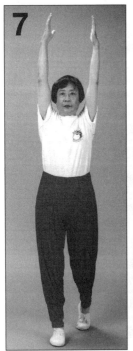
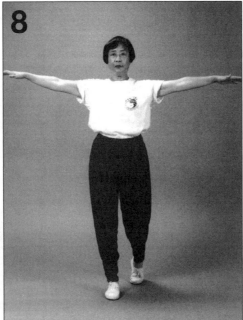
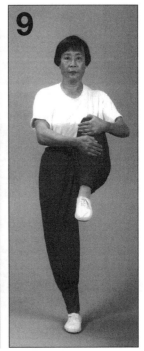

Repeat steps (1-6), but change to the right foot (7-9).

- **FREQUENCY**

  Repeat two-to-four times.

- **MAIN POINTS TO REMEMBER**

  Take only one step forward; do not go too far. Raise the arms, but do not bend the elbows.

  Stand firmly, then lift the knee up to help keep the balance.

  When holding the knee up as close to the chest as possible, keep the standing leg straight but do not lock the knee; keep the trunk erect.

- **EXERCISE SENSATIONS**

  Tension in the leg muscles.

- **BENEFITS**

  Relieves pain and stiffness in buttocks, hips and legs.

  Helps the flexion and extension of the legs.

RAMBLE THROUGH THE IMPREGNABLE PASS

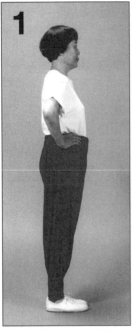

STARTING POSITION
Stand upright with feet together; place hands at the waist, thumbs pointing backward (1).

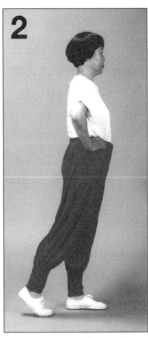

MOVEMENTS
Take a step forward with the left foot, shifting weight to the left leg and raise the right heel (2).

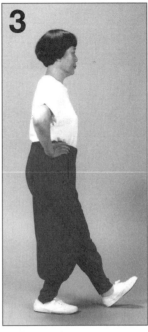

Slightly bend the right knee, shifting all the weight to the right leg and lift the sole of the left foot (3).

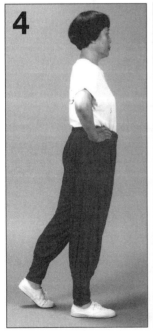

Take one step forward with the right foot, shifting weight to the right leg. Raise the left heel (4).

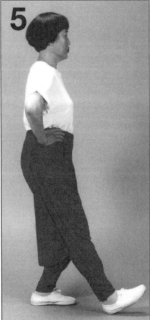

Slightly bend the left knee, shifting all the weight to the left leg. Lift the sole of the right foot (5).

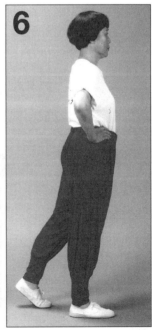

Shifting weight to the right leg, lift the left heel (6).

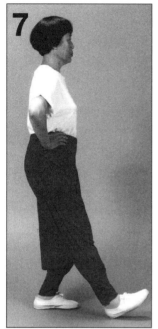
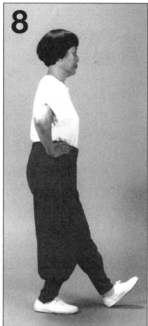
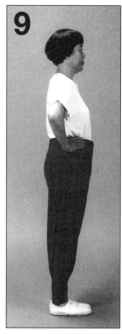

Slightly bend the left knee, shifting all the weight to the left leg. Lift the sole of the right foot (7).

Take one step backward with the right foot, shifting all the weight to the right leg. Lift the sole of the left foot (8).

Take one step backward with the left foot and return to the starting position (9). Repeat (1-9) in the opposite direction.

- **FREQUENCY**

  Repeat two-to-four times.

- **MAIN POINTS TO REMEMBER**

  Keep the torso erect, eyes looking ahead with the chest out.

  When shifting the weight forward, raise the rear heel and bend the foot until the weight of the foot is in the ball.

  When shifting the weight backward, raise the front of the toe as high as possible.

- **EXERCISE SENSATION**

  Tension in legs, ankles, and calves.

- **BENEFITS**

  Relieves pain and stiffness in the lower limbs and joints.

SECTION D
These six movements will help prevent or heal the aching joints of the four limbs.

PUSH PALMS IN HORSE STANCE

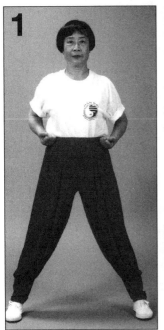
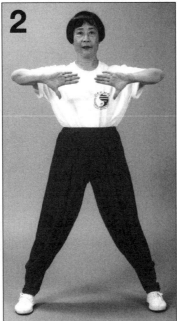
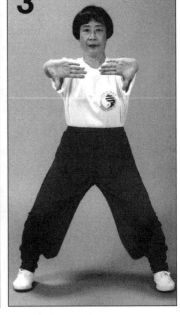

STARTING POSITION
Stand upright with the feet one and a half shoulder-widths apart. You are in a parallel stance. Your fists are at waist level (1).

MOVEMENTS
Rotate the arms at shoulder level and change the fists into palms. Keep the fingers pointing toward one another while the thumbs point down. Push the inverted palms forward; at the same time, bend the knees into a horse stance (2-3).

(Side view)   (Side view)

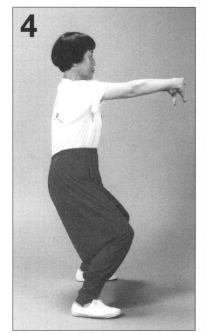
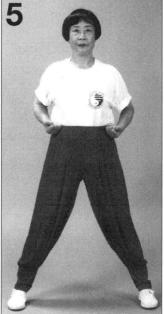
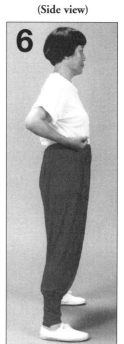

Return to the starting position (5).

- **FREQUENCY**

  Repeat two-to-four times.

- **MAIN POINTS TO REMEMBER**

  When pushing the palms forward, turn the wrists inward as much as possible and bend the wrists as far as possible. Keep the arms straight and lock the elbows.

  Do not throw the buttocks out while bending the knees into a horse stance.

  Knees are over the toes; do not extend the knees beyond the toes.

- **EXERCISE SENSATIONS**

  Tension in wrists, quadriceps and femurs of both thighs.

- **BENEFITS**

  Relieves pain in the joints of the four limbs; especially indicated for aching knees.

PUSH PALMS IN CROSS-LEG SEAT

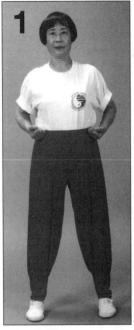
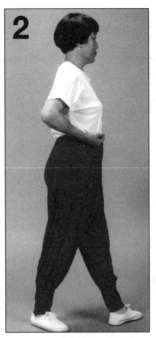
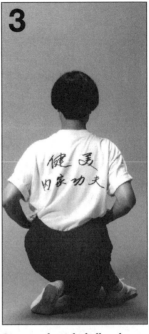

STARTING POSITION
Stand upright with the feet a shoulder-width apart. You are in a parallel stance. Your fists are at waist level (1).

MOVEMENTS
Pivot on the left heel and turn the foot 135 degrees. Pivot on the right heel and turn the foot 45 degrees (2).

Pivot on the right ball and squat down with legs crossed, the left leg over the right leg (3-4).

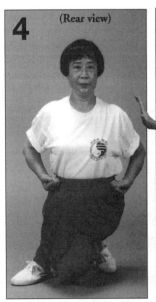
(Rear view)
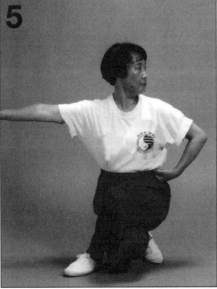
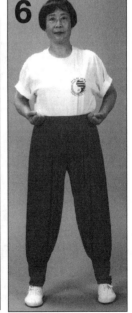

Change the right fist into a palm; push the right palm to the right, put the surface of the left fist perpendicular to your waist, palm side up, so the elbow points in the opposite direction. Turn the head to the left and look forward (5).

Stand and pivot on the right ball; turn the foot, keeping the right toe facing forward, then pivot on the left heel. Turn the foot, keeping the left toe facing forward. Return to the starting position (6-7).

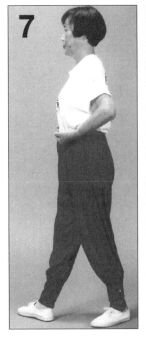 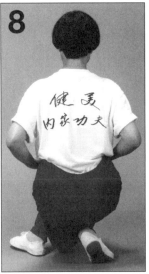 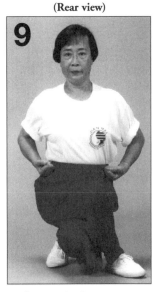

Repeat in the opposite direction (2-6).

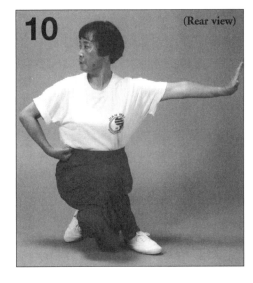

- **FREQUENCY**
  Repeat two-to-four times.
- **MAIN POINTS TO REMEMBER**
  Keep the torso upright and steady while in the cross-leg seat position.
  Pivot one foot at a time to keep balanced.
- **EXERCISE SENSATIONS**
  Tension in knees, ankles, legs and arms.
- **BENEFITS**
  Relieves aching in the arm and leg joints, neck, waist and back.

FLOW THE QI FROM TOP TO BOTTOM

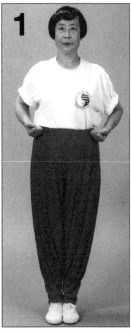
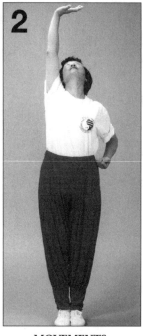
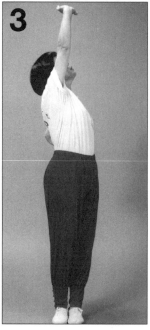

STARTING POSITION
Stand upright with feet together. You are in a parallel stance, with the fists at waist level (1).

MOVEMENTS
Change the right fist into a palm; push upward, palm facing upward, fingers pointing to the left. Look up at the back of the hand (2).

Turn the torso 90 degrees to the left (3-4).

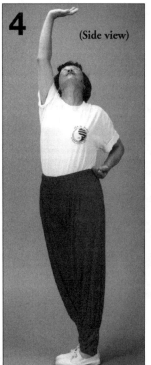
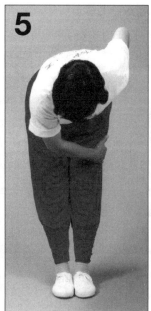
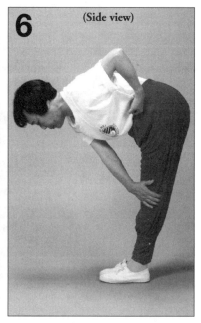

Bend the torso forward, drop the right hand to the left of the waist and slide the hand down the outside of the leg. Continue touching the top of the feet (5-7).

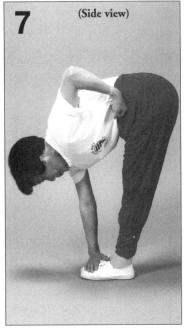
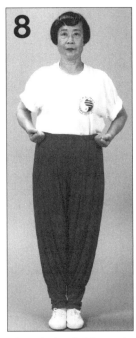
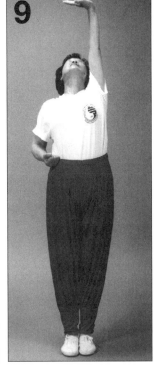

The right hand slides up the outside of the right leg, to the waist. Change the right palm into a fist and return to the starting position (8).

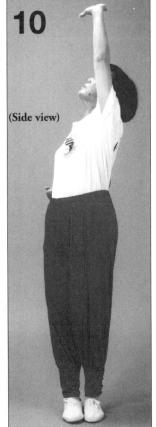
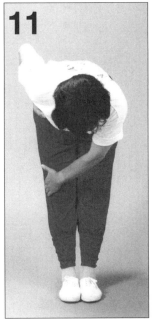
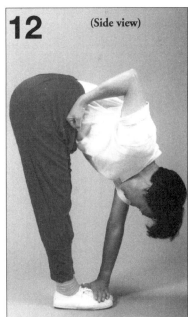

Repeat steps (2-8) in the opposite direction (9-12).

- **FREQUENCY**

  Repeat two-to-four times.

- **MAIN POINTS TO REMEMBER**

  Push the palm upward, leaving the arm close to the ear, and lock the elbow.

  Do not bend the knees while bending the torso.

- **EXERCISE SENSATIONS**

  Tension in the shoulders, arms, lower back, waist and legs.

- **FUNCTIONS**

  Relieves pain in the neck, shoulders, lower back and legs.

- **SPECIAL ADVICE**

  Cardiovascular patients: do not bend too low; keep the head higher than the heart.

TURN BODY AND HEAD

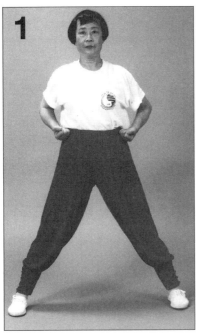

STARTING POSITION
Stand upright with the feet twice a shoulder-width apart. You are in a parallel stance, with the fists at waist level (1).

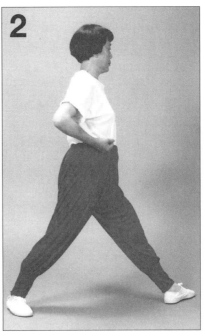

MOVEMENTS
Pivot on the left heel and turn the foot 135 degrees; pivot on the right heel and turn the foot 45 degrees (2).

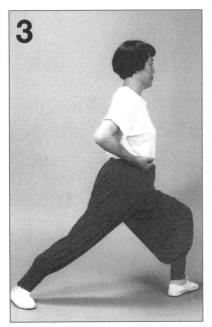

Bend the left knee into a bow stance (3).

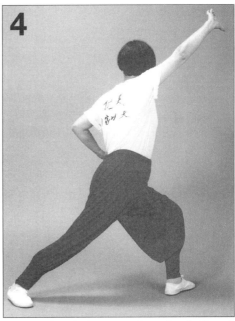

Change the right fist into a palm and push obliquely upward, twisting the right arm so the fingers are pointing left; the left elbow points backward (4).

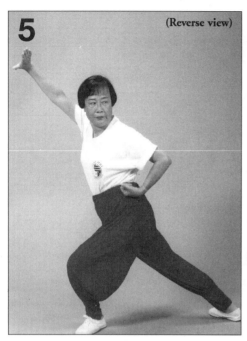
(Reverse view)

Now turn the head to look over the left shoulder (5).

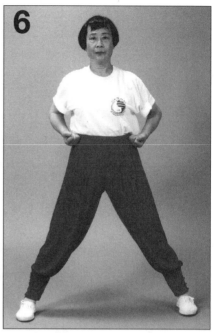

Stand. Pivot on the left heel, turn the foot and keep the left toe facing forward. Pivot on the right heel and turn the foot, keeping the right toe facing forward. Return to the starting position (1).

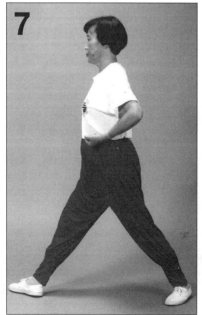

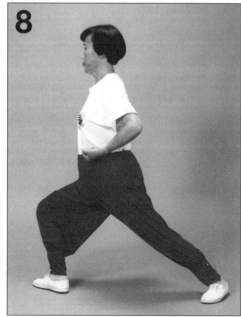

Repeat steps 1-5 but in the opposite direction (6-10).

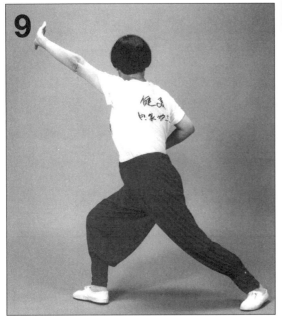
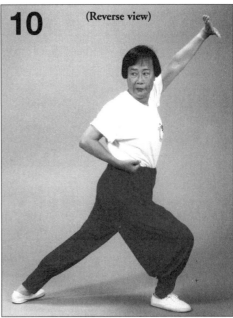

(Reverse view)

- **FREQUENCY**

  Repeat two-to-four times.

- **MAIN POINTS TO REMEMBER**

  Keep the rear leg straight; lock the knee and hold the rear foot flat on the floor while in a bow stance.

  Keep the front knee over the toe while in a bow stance.

  Push the palm obliquely upward; keep the arm in line with the leg.

  Do not lean the torso to one side.

- **EXERCISE SENSATIONS**

  Tension in the neck, shoulders, arms, lower back, waist and legs.

- **BENEFITS**

  Relieves pain in the joints of the four limbs, neck, waist and back.

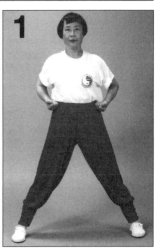

Return to the starting position (1).

HEEL KICK ON BOTH SIDES

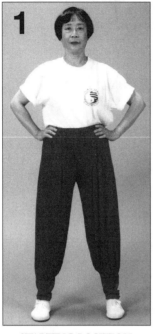

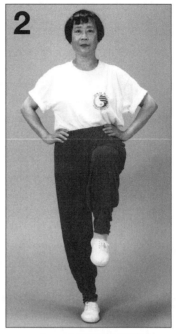

STARTING POSITION
Stand upright with the feet a shoulder-width apart. You are in a parallel stance, hands on hips, thumbs pointing backward (1).

MOVEMENTS
Lift the left knee with the toe up and stretch the left leg by kicking downward with the heel to the right (2-4).

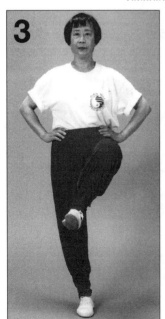

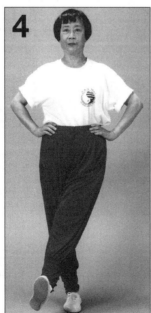

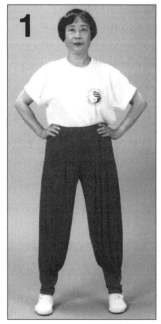

Relax the left leg; lift the left knee and return to the starting position (1).

MOVEMENTS

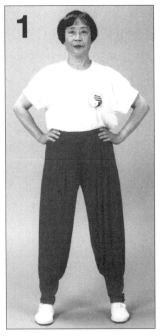

STARTING POSITION

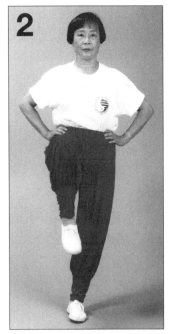

MOVEMENTS

Lift the right knee with the toe up; stretch the right leg by kicking downward with the heel to the left (2-4).

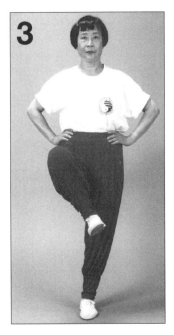

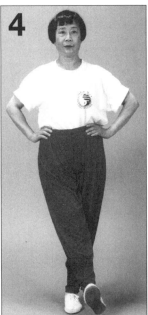

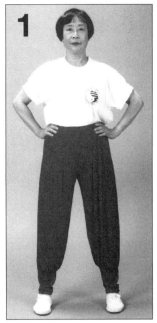

Relax the right leg; lift the right knee and return to the starting position (1).

- **FREQUENCY**

  Repeat two-to-four times.

- **MAIN POINTS TO REMEMBER**

  Remain steady when shifting weight to one leg and when lifting the knee. The other leg is straight; do not lock the knees.

  Kick down firmly with energy going through the heel.

  Keep the body erect; do not lean to one side.

- **EXERCISE SENSATIONS**

  Tension in the legs; strong tension in calves.

- **BENEFITS**

  Relieves pain in the joints and muscles of the lower limbs.

SHUTTLECOCK KICK

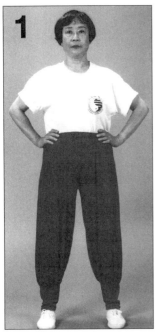
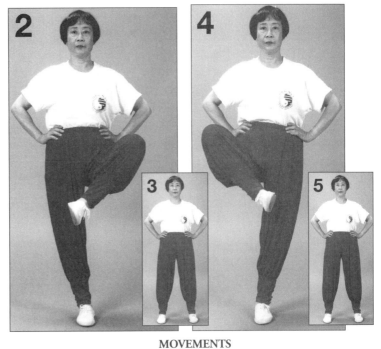

STARTING POSITION
Stand upright with the feet a shoulder-width apart. You are in a parallel stance, hands on hips and thumbs pointing backward (1).

MOVEMENTS
Left foot: Kick upward to the right with the inside of the left instep (2); return to the starting position (3). Right foot: Kick upward to the left with the inside of the right instep (4); return to the starting position (5).

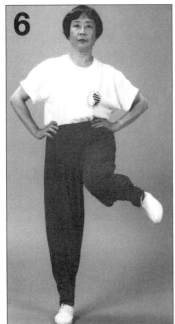
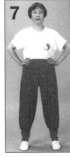
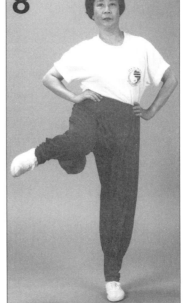
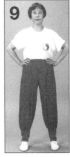

Left foot: Kick upward to the left with the outside of the left instep (6); return to the starting position (7).

Right foot: Kick upward to the right with the outside of the right instep (8); return to the starting position (9).

MOVEMENTS

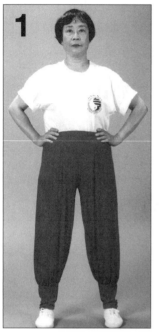

(1). STARTING POSITION

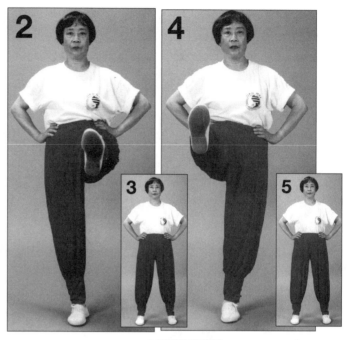

MOVEMENTS

Lift the left knee and kick forward with the toe (2); return to the starting position (3). Lift the right knee and kick forward with the toe (4); return to the starting position (5).

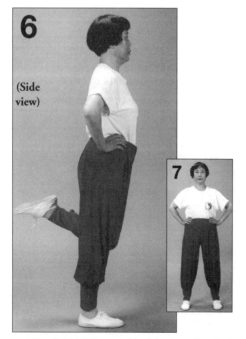

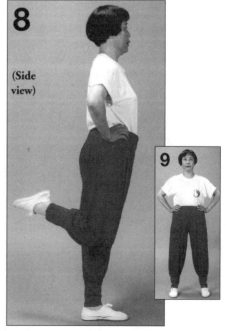

Bend the left knee and kick backward with the left heel (6); return to the starting position (7). Bend the right knee and kick backward with the right heel (8); return to the starting position (9).

- **FREQUENCY**

  Repeat two-to-four times.

- **MAIN POINTS TO REMEMBER**

  Keep the torso erect while kicking in the four directions.

  Keep the thighs perpendicular when kicking the heel toward the buttocks.

  Execute the kicks forcefully.

- **EXERCISE SENSATIONS**

  Tension in legs.

  Strong tension in the quadriceps when kicking the heel toward the buttocks.

- **BENEFITS**

  Relieves pain in the hip and knee joints.

  Strengthens the lower limbs.

SECTION E
These six movements will help you to prevent or heal injuries in the tendons and connective tissues.

PUSH PALMS IN FOUR DIRECTIONS

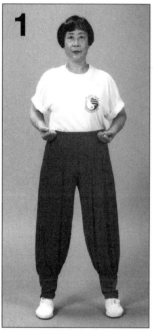
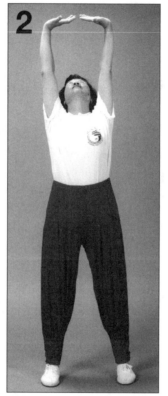
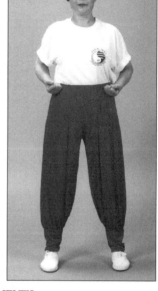

STARTING POSITION
Stand upright with your feet a shoulder-width apart. You are in a parallel stance, your fists at waist level (1).

MOVEMENTS
Change the fists into palms and push upward with the palms up. The tips of the fingers should be pointing toward one another; look at the back of the hands (2). Return to the starting position (3).

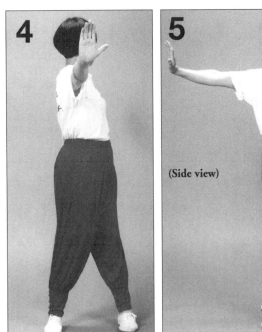
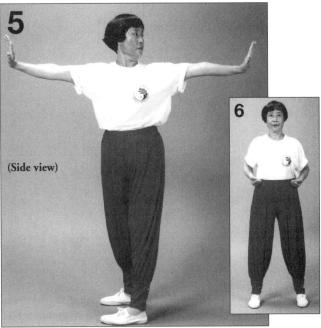

Change the fists into palms, with the tips of the fingers pointing upward. Raise the arms to shoulder level and push the palms forward and backward. At the same time, turn the torso 90 degrees to the left; the eyes look at the left hand (4-5). Return to the starting position (6).

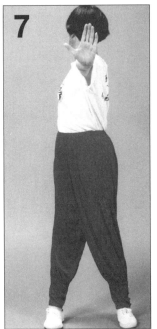
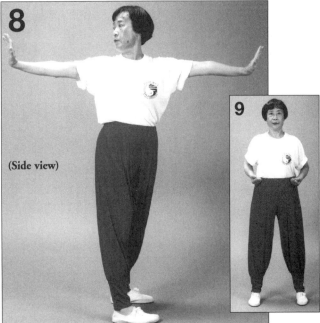

Change the fists into palms, with the tips of the fingers pointing upward. Raise the arms to shoulder level and push the palms forward and backward. At the same time, turn the torso 90 degrees to the right; the eyes look at the right hand (7-8). Return to the starting position (9).

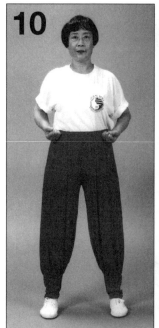
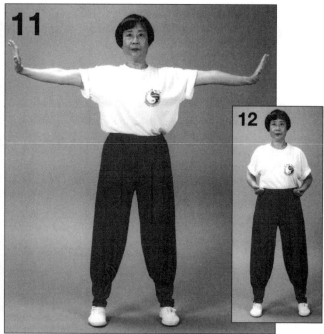

From the starting position (10), change the fists into palms, with the tips of the fingers pointing upward. Raise the arms to shoulder level and push the palms to the sides; the eyes look forward (11). Return to the starting position (12).

- **FREQUENCY**

  Repeat two-to-four times.

- **MAIN POINTS TO REMEMBER**

  Keep the torso erect and the feet flat on the ground; the feet do not move.

  Stand firm while turning the upper body.

  While pushing the palms, keep them at 90 degrees with the forearms.

- **EXERCISE SENSATIONS**

  Tension in the neck, shoulder, arms, elbows, wrists, fingers, waist, and legs.

- **BENEFITS**

  Relieves tennis elbow and tenosynovitis of the wrists and fingers.

DRAW A BOW TO SHOOT AN ARROW

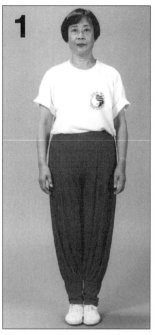
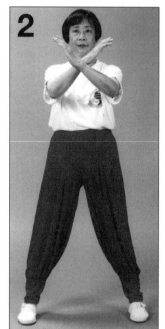
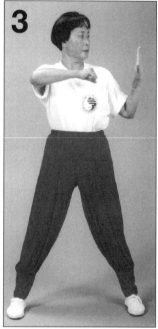

STARTING POSITION
Relax the body; keep the body erect, feet together and arms at your sides. The eyes look forward (1).

MOVEMENTS
Move the left foot to the left, one and a half shoulder-widths apart. You are in a parallel stance. At the same time, cross the palms at the wrists in front of the chest (about 10-to-12 inches), with the left outside (2). Change the right palm into a fist and the left palm to the left shoulder level. The tips of the fingers are pointing upward (3).

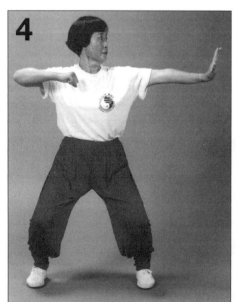
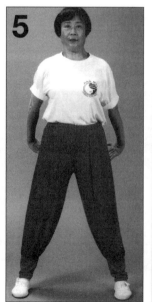
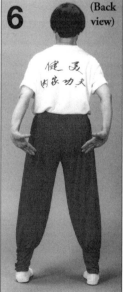

(Back view)

Push the left palm to the left and pull the right fist in front of the right shoulder; the eyes look at the left hand. At the same time, bend the knees into a horse stance (4).

Open the right fist into a palm and press the palms backward and downward. The tips of the fingers point to one another with the elbows locked; lock the knees and stretch the legs (5-6).

MOVEMENTS

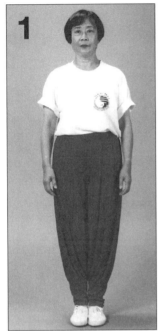
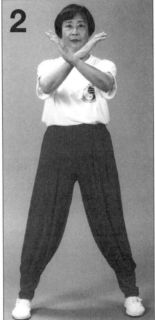
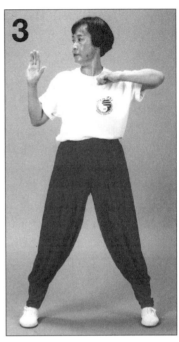

Return to the starting position (1). Same as steps 2-6, but in the opposite direction (2-6).

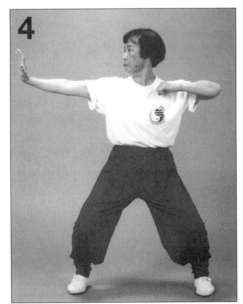
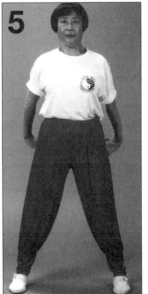
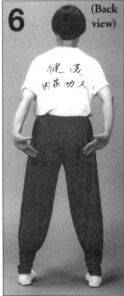

Push the right palm to the right and pull the left fist in front of the left shoulder; the eyes look at the right hand. At the same time, bend the knees into a horse stance (4).

Open the left fist into a palm and press the palms backward and downward. The tips of the fingers point to one another with the elbows locked; lock the knees and stretch the legs (5-6). Return to the starting position.

- **FREQUENCY**

  Repeat two-to-four times.

- **MAIN POINTS TO REMEMBER**

  Do not throw the buttocks out while bending the knees into a horse stance.

  Keep the palm at 90 degrees with the forearms while extending them.

  When pulling the fist and pushing the palm, the elbow and palm point in opposite directions. Keep the arms and fists at shoulder level.

  Throw the chest out while performing steps 5-6; squeeze the shoulder blades as close as possible to the spine.

- **EXERCISE SENSATIONS**

  Tension in the forearms, wrists, fingers, neck, back and quadriceps.

- **BENEFITS**

  Relieves tennis elbow and tenosynovitis of the wrists, fingers and toes.

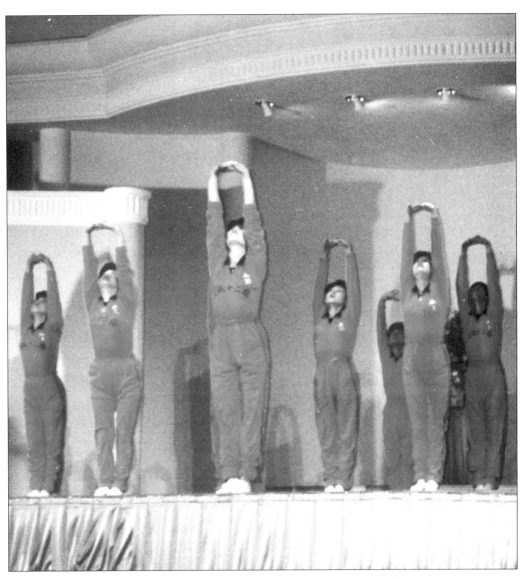

Liangong demonstration at the 1992 International Conference in Shanghai, China.

STRETCH ARMS AND TURN WRISTS

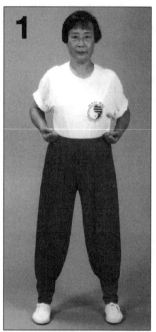
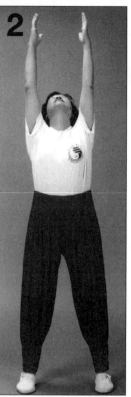
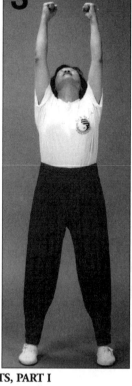

STARTING POSITION
Stand upright with the feet a shoulder-width apart. You are in a parallel stance, with the fists at waist level.(1).

MOVEMENTS, PART I
Change the fists into palms; stretch upward with the palms facing each other and the eyes looking upward (2) and change the palms into fists (3).

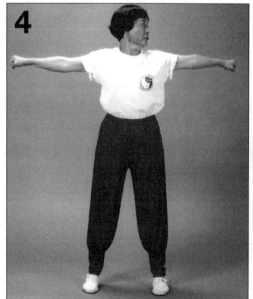
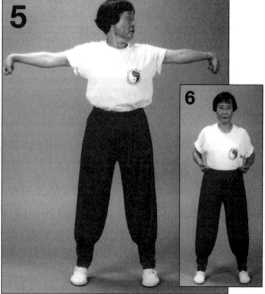

Drop and rotate them to the sides and back as far as possible; bend the wrists while the arms drop to shoulder level; the eyes follow the left hand (4-5). Then slightly bend the elbows and return to the starting position (6). Repeat steps 1-6, but in the opposite direction.

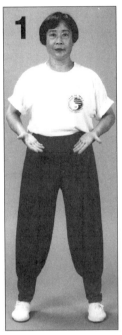 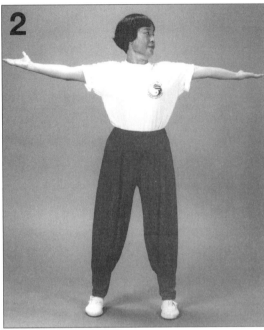 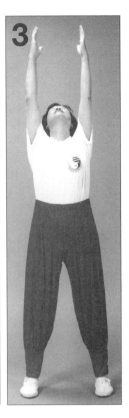

MOVEMENTS, PART II

Change the fists into palms; stretch downward and backward with palms facing upward while the arms rise to shoulder level. The eyes follow the left hand (1-2) Continue to raise the palms upward over the head with the palms facing each other. The eyes look upward (3).

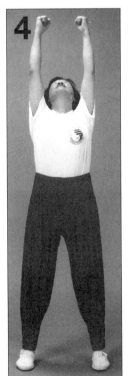 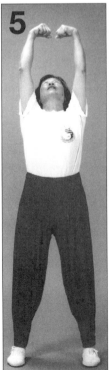 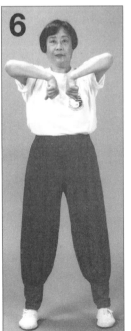

Change the palms into fists (4). Bend the wrists inward (5); pull the fists down and slightly bend the elbow. Keep the back of the fists facing each other (6), and return to the starting position (7).

Repeat steps 1-7, with step 2 in the opposite direction.

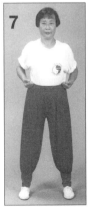

- **FREQUENCY**

  Repeat two-to-four times.

- **MAIN POINTS TO REMEMBER**

  Stretch the arms upward; keep the arms straight, lock the elbows, and stand with the feet a shoulder-width apart.

  Continually bend the wrists inward while pulling the fist down.

  Throw the chest out while stretching.

- **EXERCISE SENSATIONS**

  Tension in the wrists, elbows, shoulder and arms.

- **BENEFITS**

  Relieves soreness and stiffness of rheumatic shoulders, tennis elbow, and tenosynovitis of wrists and fingers.

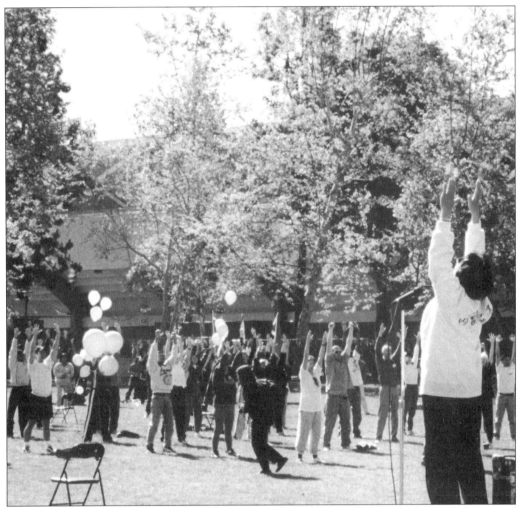

Liangong at First World Tai Chi Day at UCLA, in Westwood, Calif.

EXTEND ARMS FORWARD AND BACKWARD

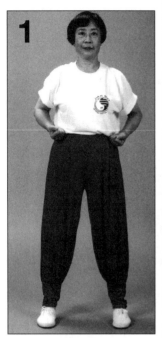
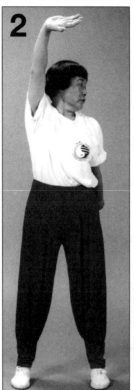
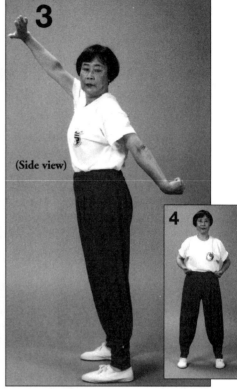

(Side view)

STARTING POSITION
Stand upright, with the feet a shoulder-width apart. You are in a parallel stance, with the fists at waist level (1)

MOVEMENTS
Change the right fist into a palm; push obliquely upward and forward with the fingers pointing left and the thumb pointing downward. At the same time, turn the left fist inward; bend the wrist and stretch it obliquely downward and backward with the back of the fist facing downward (2-3). The eyes look at the left fist. Return to the starting position (4).

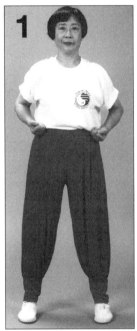 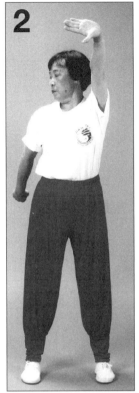 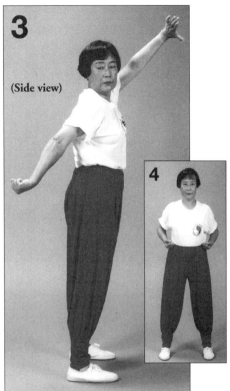

From the starting position (1), change the left fist into a palm; push obliquely upward and forward with the fingers pointing right, thumb pointing downward. At the same time, turn the right fist inward; bend the wrist and stretch it obliquely downward and backward with the back of the fist facing downward. The eyes look at the right fist (2-3). Return to the starting position (4).

- **FREQUENCY**

  Repeat two-to-four times.

- **MAIN POINTS TO REMEMBER**

  Keep the palm 90 degrees with the forearms while pushing the palm.

  Keep the front and back arms in a straight line; lock the elbows.

  Do not turn the torso; turn the head only, and keep the shoulders square.

- **EXERCISE SENSATIONS**

  Tension in the shoulders, arms, elbows, wrists, and fingers as well as chest.

- **BENEFITS**

  Relieves pain and stiffness in the shoulders, and eases tennis elbow and tenosynovitis of the wrist and fingers.

  Effective in preventing and treating lower back pain.

PUNCH IN HORSE STANCE

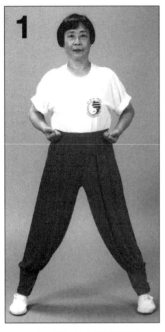
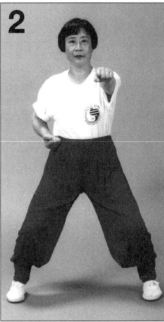
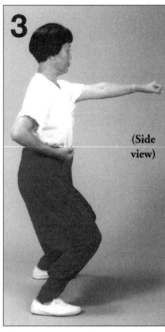

STARTING POSITION
Stand upright with the feet one and a half shoulder-widths apart. You are in a parallel stance, with the fists at waist level (1).

MOVEMENTS
Raise the left fist and punch forward with the back of the fist facing upward. At the same time, bend the knees into a horse stance (2-3).

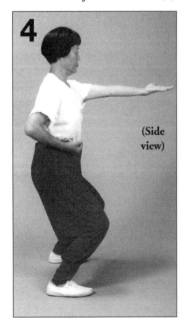
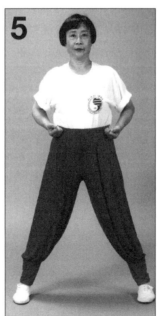
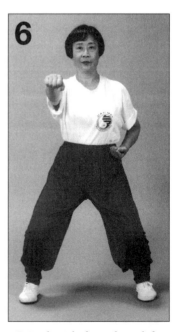

Open the left fist and turn the palm upward (4). Gradually change the left palm into a fist and return to the starting position (5).

Raise the right fist and punch forward with the back of the fist facing upward. At the same time, bend the knees into a horse stance (6).

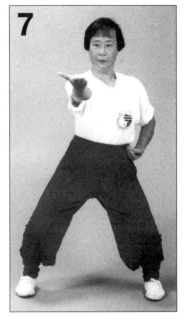 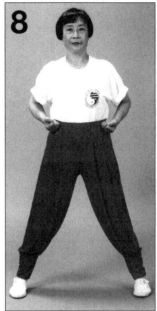

Open the right fist and turn the palm upward (7), gradually changing the right palm into a fist and returning to the starting position (8).

- **FREQUENCY**

  Repeat two-to-four times.

- **MAIN POINTS TO REMEMBER**

  Do not throw the buttocks out while bending the knees into a horse stance.

  Keep the shoulders square while punching; fist and shoulder are in one straight line. Do not bend the wrists.

  The fist punches forcibly using internal power.

  Stretch the palm and thumb when turning the palm upward.

- **EXERCISE SENSATIONS**

  Tension in arms, shoulders, legs, palms and thumbs.

- **BENEFITS**

  Relieves pain in the shoulders, and eases tennis elbow and tenosynovitis of wrists and fingers.

  Relieves pain and stiffness in knees, hips and lower back.

RELAX ARMS AND TURN WAIST

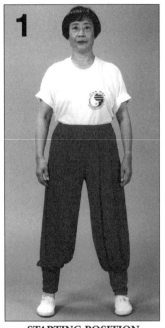

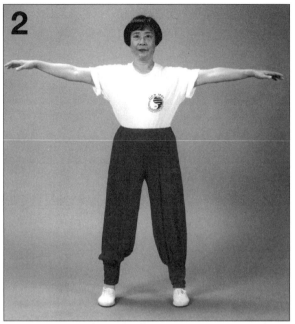

STARTING POSITION
Stand upright with the feet a shoulder-width apart. You are in a parallel stance, with the arms at your sides. The eyes are looking forward (1).

MOVEMENTS
Relax and raise the arms to shoulder level (2).

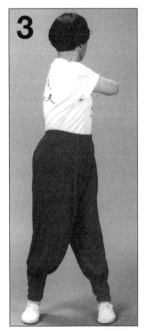

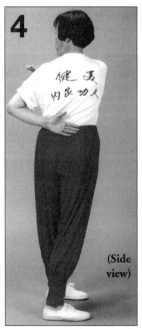

(Side view)

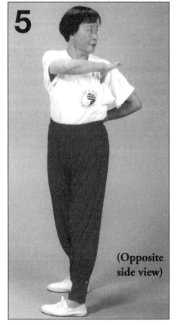

(Opposite side view)

Turn the torso 90 degrees to the left and swing the arms. Put the right thumb and forefinger of the right hand on the left shoulder, the palm facing outward. At the same time, put the back of the left hand on the lower back (mingmen point). Look backward (3-5).

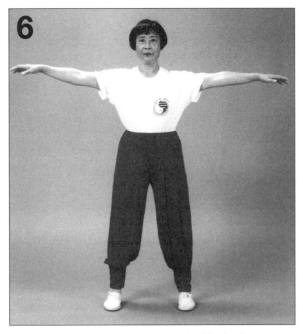

Relax and raise the arms to shoulder level (6)

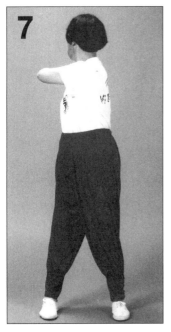
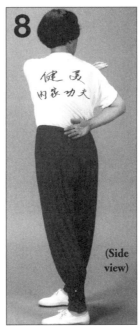
(Side view)
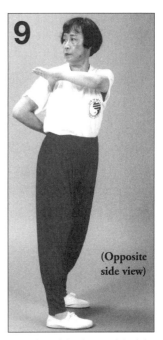
(Opposite side view)

Turn the torso 90 degrees to the right and swing the arms. Put the left thumb and forefinger of the left hand on the right shoulder, with the palm facing outward. At the same time, put the back of the right hand on the lower back (mingmen point); look backward (7-9).

- **FREQUENCY**

  Repeat two-to-four times.

- **MAIN POINTS TO REMEMBER**

  Keep the torso upright; do not lean in any direction.

  Keep the weight centered and the feet flat on the ground while turning the torso 90 degrees to the left or right.

  Relax the arms and shoulders while swinging.

  When finished swinging the arms, keep the forearms at shoulder level.

- **EXERCISE SENSATIONS**

  Tension in neck, shoulders, elbows, wrists, fingers, waist, and legs.

- **BENEFITS**

  Relieves tennis elbow, pain and stiffness in a frozen shoulder, waist and lower back.

SECTION F
These six movements will help you prevent or heal internal disorders.

MASSAGE FACE AND ACUPRESSURE POINTS

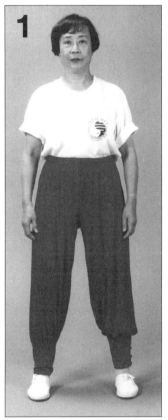

STARTING POSITION
Stand upright with the feet a shoulder-width apart. You are in a parallel stance, with the arms at your sides. Look forward (1).

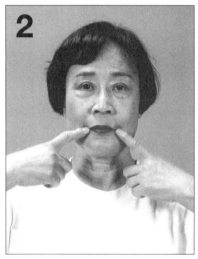

MOVEMENTS
Massage the face using the index fingertips from Di-cang (2) upward, through Ying-xiang (3).

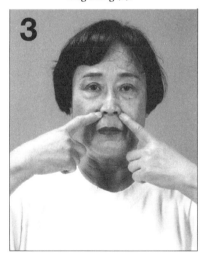

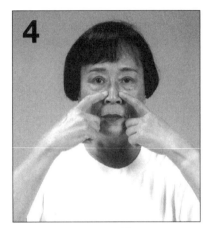
Bi-tong (4).

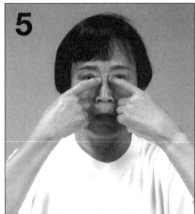
Jing-ming (5).

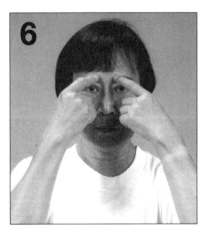
Zan-zhu (6).

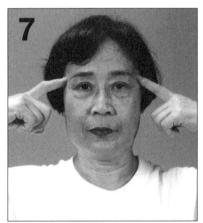
Tai-yang (7).

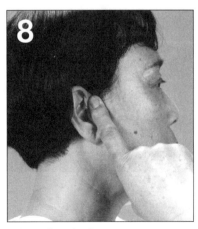
Move the index fingertips, crossing over Er-men (8).

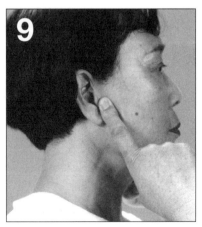
Ting-gong and Ting-hui (9).
Massage eight-to-16 times.

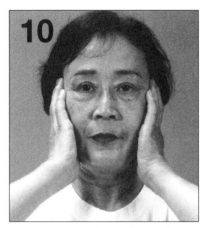

Massage the face with the palms from the jaw (10)...

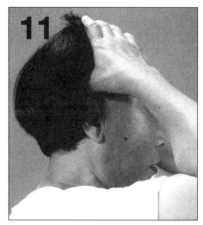

...upward to the top of head (11).

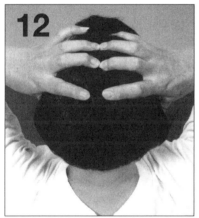

The middle fingers pressure the acupoint Bai-hui (12).

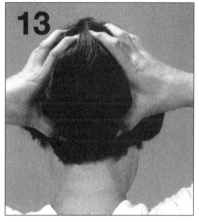

Move the thumbs to acupoint Feng-chi (13);

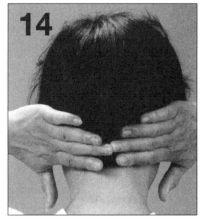

knead several times (14),

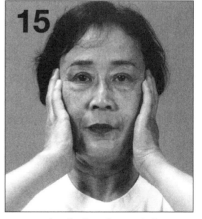

then back to the jaw (15). Massage eight-to-16 times.

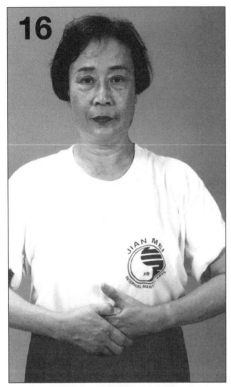
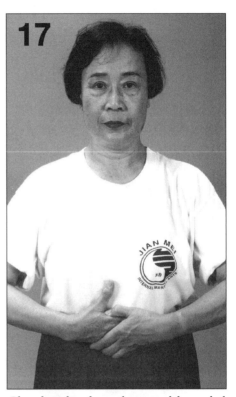

Place the left palm on the upper abdomen; look forward and grasp the left hand with the right hand. The right thumb kneads acupoint Shui-mian on the left hand (16).
Massage back and forth 32 times.

Place the right palm on the upper abdomen; look forward and grasp the right hand with the left hand. The left thumb kneads acupoint Shui-mian on the right hand (17).
Massage back and forth 32 times.

- **MAIN POINTS TO REMEMBER**

  When massaging the acupoints, use the tips of the fingers and apply pressure while kneading.

  Close the eyes and empty the mind when kneading the Shui-mian point.

- **EXERCISE SENSATIONS**

  Warmth on the face. Soreness while kneading all the acupoints.

- **BENEFITS**

  Relieves nervousness, insomnia, dizziness, palpitation of the heart and stomach, and intestinal disorders.

MASSAGE CHEST AND ABDOMEN

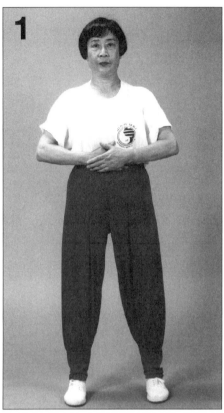

STARTING POSITION
Stand upright with the feet a shoulder-width apart. You are in a parallel stance, with the palms on the upper abdomen, left palm on top of right palm (1).

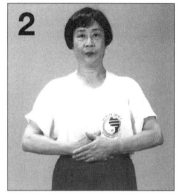

MOVEMENTS
Massage the upper abdomen in clockwise circles eight times (2).

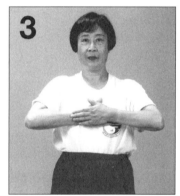

Enlarge the clockwise circle from the chest to the lower abdomen and massage eight times (3).

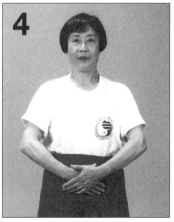

Massage from the chest to the lower abdomen counterclockwise eight times (4).

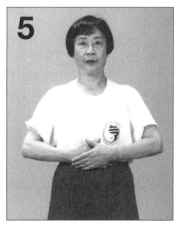

Massage the upper abdomen in counterclockwise circles eight times (5).

- **FREQUENCY**

  Repeat two-to-four times.

- **MAIN POINTS TO REMEMBER**

  Exert some internal force (nei-jing).

  Eyes look straight ahead.

  Relax the abdomen.

- **EXERCISE SENSATIONS**

  Warmth in abdomen; belching followed by a feeling of relief and a comfortable, smooth feeling when you hiccup.

- **BENEFITS**

  Relieves functional disorders of the stomach and intestines.

COMB HAIR AND TURN WAIST

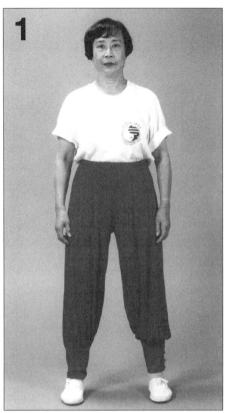

STARTING POSITION
Stand upright with the feet a shoulder-width apart. You are in a parallel stance, with the arms at your sides. Look forward (1).

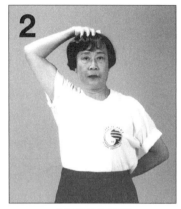

MOVEMENTS
Place the right palm on top of the head, fingers pointing forward (2). At the same time, place the back of the left hand on the Ming-men acupoint.

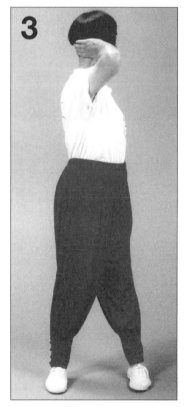

Turn the torso 90 degrees to the left and turn the head 180 degrees, with the eyes looking backward; at the same time, comb the hair backward with four fingers of the right hand to the occipital bone (3).

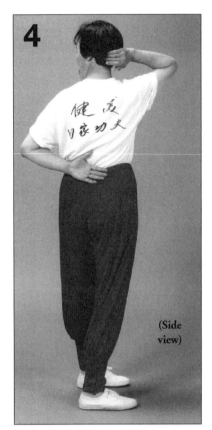
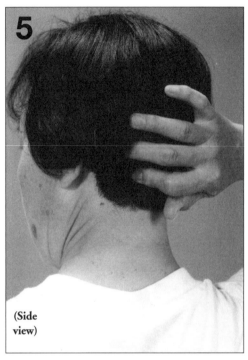

(Side view)

(Side view)

Knead the left Feng-chi point (4-5)

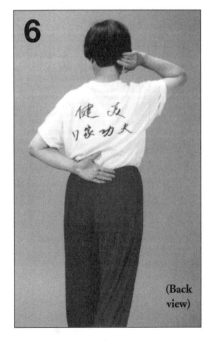
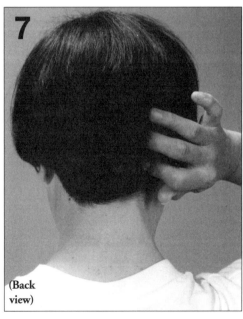

(Back view)

(Back view)

and then knead the right Feng-chi point (6-7).

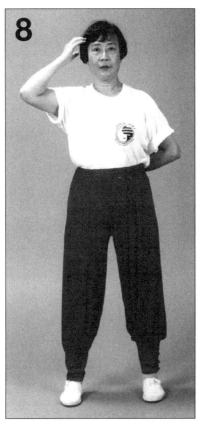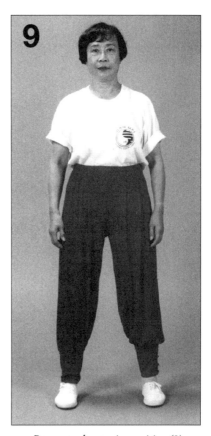

Turn the torso forward. At the same time, move the fingers from the right Feng-chi to the right Shuai-gu acupoint. Massage several times (8).

Return to the starting position (9).

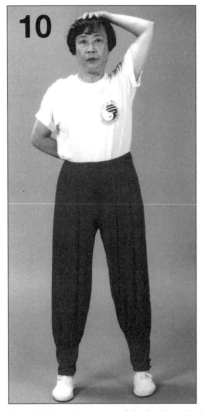
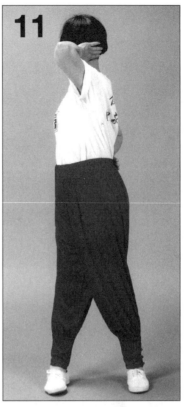

Place the left palm on top of the head, with the fingers pointing forward (10). At the same time, place the back of the right hand on the Ming-men acupoint.

Turn the torso 90 degrees to the right and turn the head 180 degrees, with the eyes looking backward; at the same time, comb the hair backward with the four fingers of the left hand to the occipital bone (11).

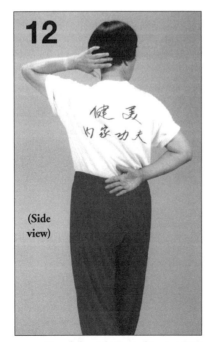
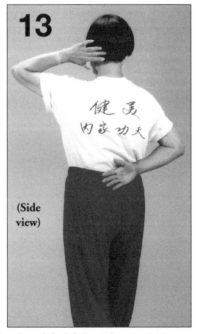

Knead the right Feng-chi point (12) and then knead the left Feng-chi point (13).

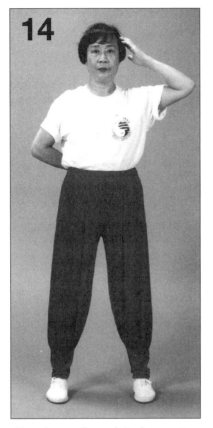
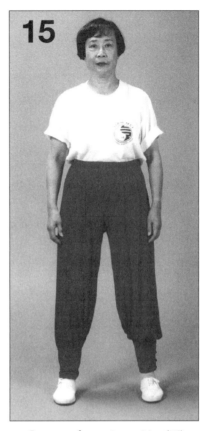

Turn the torso forward. At the same time, move the fingers from the left Feng-chi to the left Shuai-gu acupoint. Massage several times (14).

Return to the starting position (15).

- **FREQUENCY**

  Repeat two-to-four times.

- **MAIN POINTS TO REMEMBER**

  Press the palm firmly on the head and exert force (nei-jing) while combing.

  Keep the torso straight. When turning the torso, do not shift your weight.

  The movements must be slow, continuous, and gradual.

- **EXERCISE SENSATIONS**

  The head feels relaxed and comfortable.

  Tension in the waist.

- **BENEFITS**

  Relieves dizziness, blurred vision, insomnia and palpitation.

  Relieves headaches.

HOLD UP PALM AND LIFT KNEE

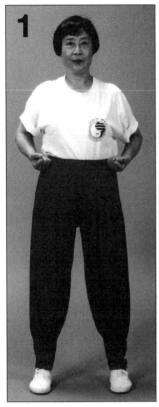

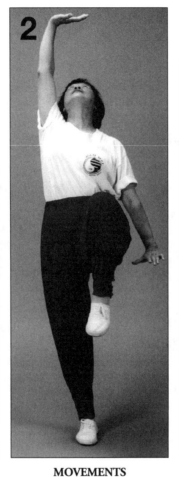

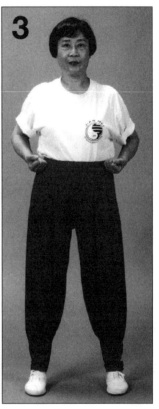

STARTING POSITION
Stand upright with the feet a shoulder-width apart. You are in a parallel stance, with the fists at waist level (1).

MOVEMENTS
Shifting weight onto the right foot, raise the right palm upward over the head. The arm is close to the ear, the fingers point left, and the eyes look at the back of the right hand. At the same time, change the left fist to a palm and push downward. The fingers point forward. Lift the left knee as high as possible (2).

Return to the starting position (3).

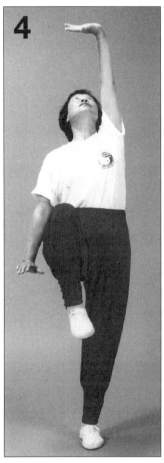
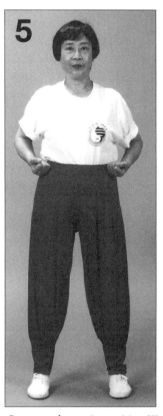

Shifting weight onto the left foot, raise the left palm upward over the head. The arm is close to the ear, the fingers point right, and the eyes look at the back of the left hand. At the same time, change the right fist to a palm and push downward, fingers pointing forward. Lift the right knee as high as possible (4).

Return to the starting position (5).

- **FREQUENCY**

  Repeat two-to-four times.

- **MAIN POINTS TO REMEMBER**

  Keep the torso straight; stretch the arms as far as possible.

  Lift the knees as high as possible; relax the leg and let the lower leg hang; stand steadily on one leg.

- **EXERCISE SENSATIONS**

  Tension in the neck, shoulders, arms, back and legs.

  Relaxed feeling in the chest and abdomen.

- **BENEFITS**

  Strengthens the spleen and stomach, improving digestion.

TURN AND BEND BODY

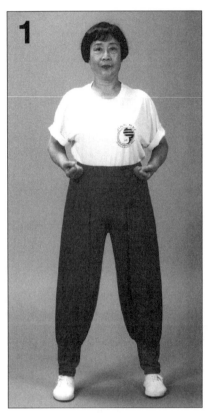

STARTING POSITION
Stand upright with the feet a shoulder-width apart. You are in a parallel stance, with the fists at waist level (1).

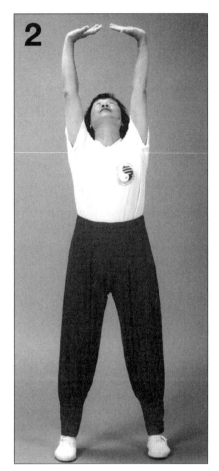

MOVEMENTS
Change the fists to palms; push the palms upward over the head, fingers pointing at one another. The eyes look at the back of the hands (2).

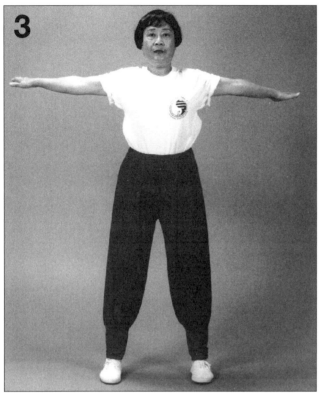
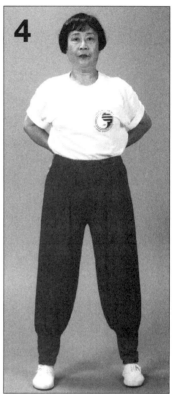

Drop the palms down sideways (3); place the palms on the waist, fingers pointing downward and thumbs pointing forward (4-5).

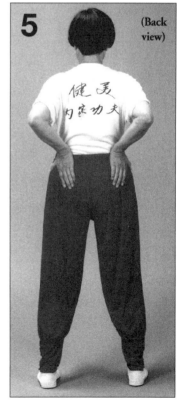

(Back view)

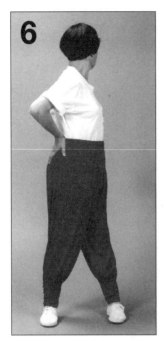
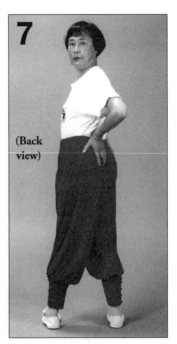

*Turn the torso to the left as far as possible;
the eyes look backward (6-7).*

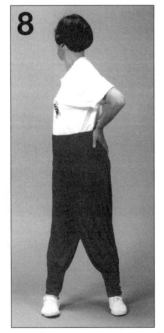
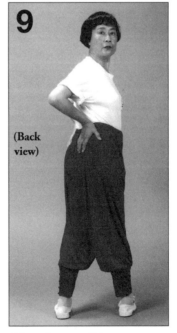

*Turn the torso to the right as far as possible;
the eyes look backward (8-9).*

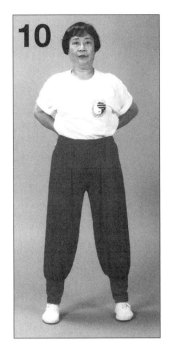
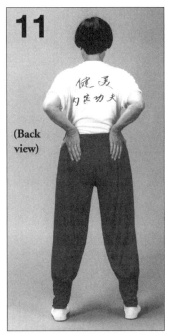

Turn the torso forward, the eyes look forward (10-11).

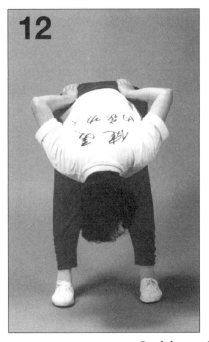
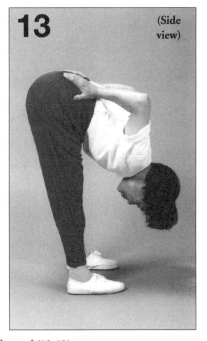

Bend the torso forward (12-13).

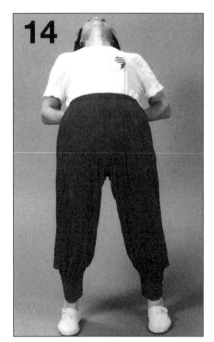 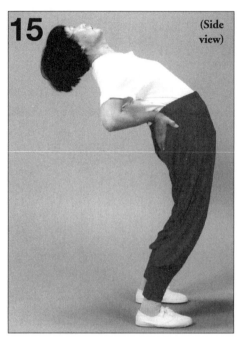

Raise the torso and bend backward (14-15).

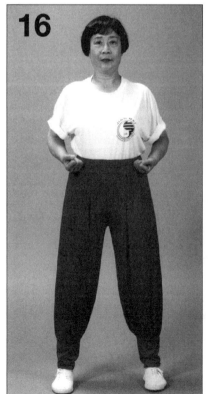

Return to the starting position (16).

- **FREQUENCY**

  Repeat two-to-four times.

- **MAIN POINTS TO REMEMBER**

  When dropping the palms sideways, reach back as far as possible.

  Keep the feet flat on the ground when turning the torso to the left or to the right. Stand firmly.

  Turn the torso to the left or right at least 90 degrees; turn the head 180 degrees, keeping the torso erect.

  Keep the legs straight; lock the knees when turning or bending.

  Do not bend the neck forward or backward when bending.

  Stand firmly; do not lose balance when bending backward.

- **EXERCISE SENSATIONS**

  Tension in the neck, arms, shoulders, waist and legs.

- **BENEFITS**

  Relieves pain in the neck, shoulders, waist and back.

  Improves kidney deficiencies, recovery time from fatigue, and strengthens the constitution.

- **SPECIAL ADVICE**

  Cardiovascular patients: do not bend forward too low; keep the head higher than the heart.

EXTEND ARMS AND SPREAD CHEST

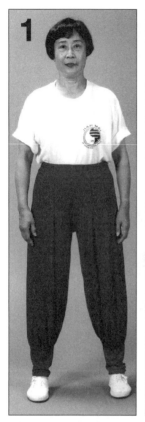
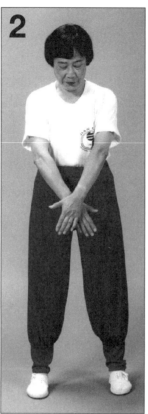
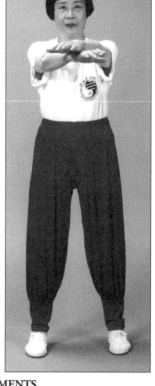

STARTING POSITION
Stand upright with the feet a shoulder-width apart. You are in a parallel stance, with the arms at your side. Look forward (1).

MOVEMENTS
Stack the hands in front of the lower abdomen (left on top) and raise them upward from the front (2-3).

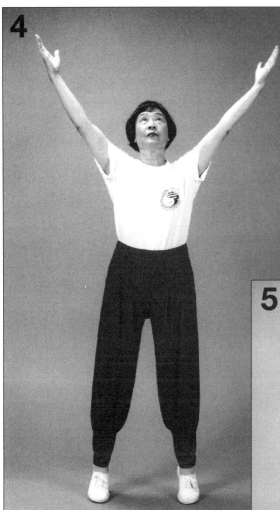

Separate the hands with the fingers pointing obliquely upward above the head to form a "V." At the same time, lift the heels and inhale deeply (4-5).

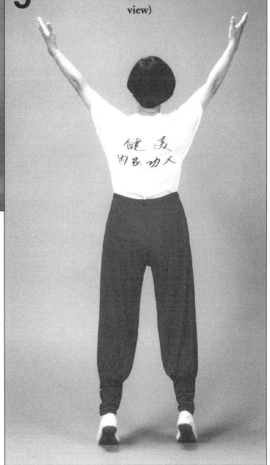

(Back view)

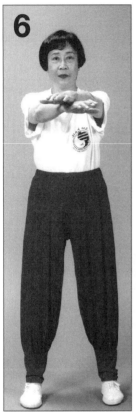
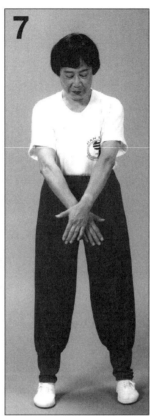
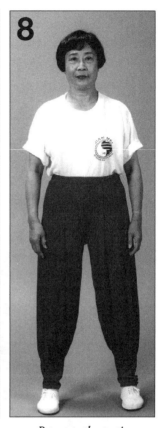

Drop the hands from the front and stack them (left on top) in front of the lower abdomen (6-7).

Return to the starting position. At the same time, lower the heels and exhale (8).

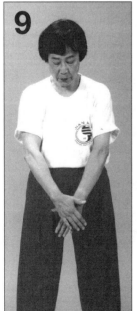
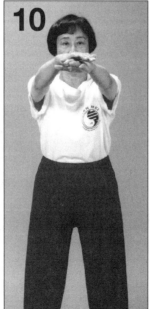

Stack the hands in front of the lower abdomen (right on top) and raise them upward from the front (9-10).

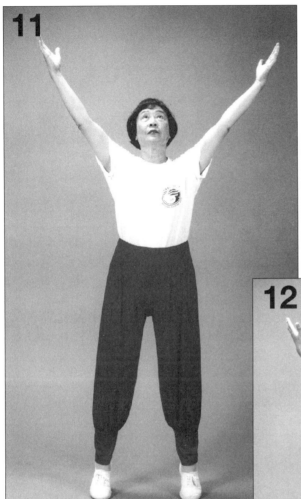

Separate the hands with the fingers pointing obliquely upward above the head to form a "V." At the same time, lift the heels and inhale deeply (11-12).

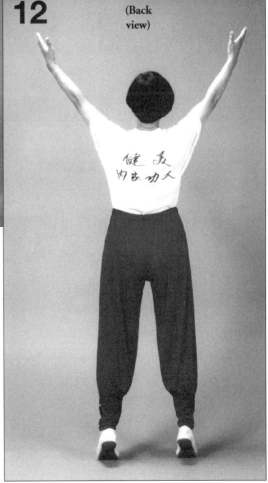

(Back view)

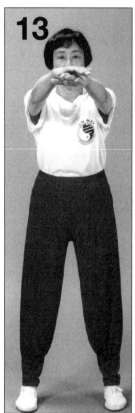 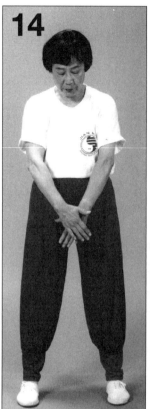 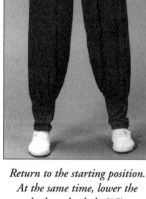

Drop the hands from the front and stack them (right on top) in front of the lower abdomen (13-14).

Return to the starting position. At the same time, lower the heels and exhale (15).

- **FREQUENCY**

  Repeat two-to-four times.

- **MAIN POINTS TO REMEMBER**

  Do not separate the hands before they have been raised above the head.

  First, shift all the weight to the balls of the feet, then lift the heels. It will help you maintain balance.

  When forming the "V," the eyes look obliquely forward. Do not bend the neck.

- **EXERCISE SENSATIONS**

Combining deep breathing with the movements results in a comfortable and pleasant feeling in the chest.

- **BENEFITS**

Relieves chronic diseases of the respiratory and digestive systems.

Closing position. Relax. Keep the body erect, feet together, arms at your sides, and eyes looking forward.

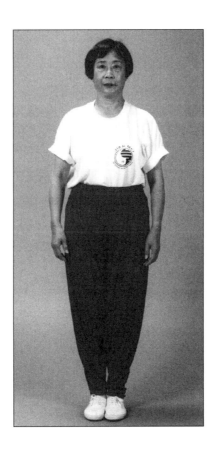

Chapter 7

TESTIMONIALS

A MASTER'S MASTER

Every Wednesday morning rain or shine, Wen-Mei Yu leaves her suburban Los Angeles home and makes a 45-minute trek south along the 405 to the city of Westwood and the campus of UCLA.

It is there among the scholars of today and the leaders of tomorrow that Master Yu brings peace and hope to people young and old suffering from the effects of cancer. Although her Guo Lin Chi Kung exercise regimen lasts about an hour, the difference her words, and more importantly her actions, bring to the 20-to-30 in her group is immeasurable. She is giving those sufferers hope. She is giving them time. She is giving them comfort.

Master Yu doesn't do it for the money. She doesn't do it for the notoriety. She doesn't do it for the publicity. She shares the healing powers of chi kung because it makes her feel good to know she's making others feel better.

There are reports out of China that a regimen of tai chi and chi kung has been known to slow and in some cases even stop cancer's deadly run through the body. Master Yu has read the studies and knows the power chi kung can have on someone who's resistance is woefully lacking. As one who witnessed first hand the curative powers of chi kung, Master Yu has come to appreciate what the internal arts mean to those with nowhere else to turn.

In a time of self-made masters and overnight sifu, Master Wen-Mei Yu is a genuine original. Her pedigree reads like a who's who of internal arts mastery. Consider the physicist who studied under Einstein. The painter who carried the brushes of Van Gough. Or the architect who learned to draw at the hands of Frank Lloyd Wright. The names on her resume are among the finest and most-respected internal arts masters the martial arts world has ever known.

Wu Ying Hua. Ma Yueh Liang. Fu Zhong Wen. Gu Liu Xin. Zhou Yuan Long. Guo Ling. Dr. Zhuang Yuan Ming. Zhao Jin Xiang. These aren't just footnotes in the history of internal martial arts. These are giants credited with creating some of the finest and most-complete exercise systems ever devised.

Master Yu came to the United States in 1987 at a time when the Western world was hungry for authentic tai chi instruction. Proving her worth in many of the most-prestigious tournaments, she quickly became a respected and sought-after authority on the benefits of tai chi and chi kung training. Fifteen years of seminars, demonstrations and performances have only proven what those in her native China knew all along: she is one of our living treasures — a martial artist whose knowledge is so great, whose heart is so deep that many of her contributions will only be felt long after she is gone.

I have known Master Wen-Mei Yu for 15 years and consider her not only a great friend, but one of the finest and most generous individuals in martial arts. Her ability to teach, to communicate, to bring internal arts to the masses is virtually unmatched in today's society.

The book you hold in your hand today is the first of what I hope to be many written by one of our finest masters and greatest teachers. I hope you enjoy reading it as much as I have enjoyed getting to know its author.

— Dave Cater
Editor, *Inside Kung-Fu*

LIANGONG

*O*ver the years I have been involved in many sports: golf, tennis, skiing, volleyball, aerobics, weight training, and tai chi. Invariably I have injured my shoulder, knees, ankles, wrist, groin, hamstrings, back, etc. Many of these injuries were a result of tight muscles and joints, and improper body alignment. Two years ago, I learned Liangong from Master Yu. What I found is that Liangong provides a good strategy for preventing injuries, and provides a quicker recovery when injured.

The systematic exercises insure that all the major muscles, joints, and tendons from head to toe are gently stretched with movements that specifically target these vulnerable areas. Since practicing Liangong, my flexibility and strength have increased in my arms, legs, and back. It has been very encouraging to see these positive changes in my body.

Pam Dong, Ph.D.
Pasadena, CA

*A*fter taking Master Yu's Liangong class my whole body felt stretched, relaxed and strong. I am now using these exercises in the tai chi classes I teach as I feel they "do the job" as an excellent warm-up.

Roxanne Chappell
Vancouver, B.C., Canada
Director of Women's Festival
Of Martial Arts

*I*n 1993 I went to the National Women's Martial Arts Summer Training Camp in New York. I was bothered with a lump in my shoulder due to calcium deposits, and was going to have surgery after the training camp was over. There I met Master Yu who was teaching Liangong, and she suggested that I give these exercises a try. After two days of practicing Liangong the lump had already reduced in size. I postponed the surgery and continued to do Liangong. After a few months, the lump completely disappeared and I was able to avoid surgery completely.

Virginia Bunside
Caledonia, NY

TESTIMONIALS

Caledonia, NY

My body likes Liangong. It's very good for getting to areas that haven't been touched for a long time, meaning you can feel where your body is stuck. The energy that Liangong utilizes opens these stuck places and you feel a warm pulsing. I have had so many injuries in my life that restrict my movements when playing golf, but I have found that just doing the elemental movements of Liangong have allowed me freedom of movement that I did not have.

Craig T. Nelson
Malibu, CA

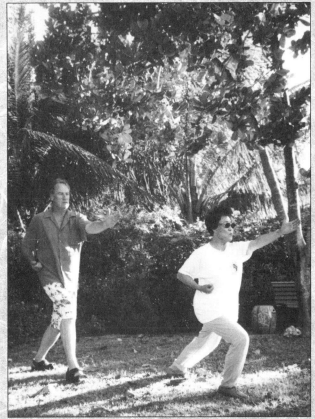

With over 20 years of involved taiji/qigong practice, I first learned Liangong from Master Yu believing it to simply be a rejuvenating exercise designed mainly for the general public. But after four years of applying it to my personal warm-ups and teaching programs, Liangong has revealed itself to be multifaceted and significantly effective, even for those who generally dislike exercise.

Feedback from my students (especially Western doctors and the physically challenged) and routine discussions with taiji/acupuncture colleagues continually reaffirms how cleverly these movements have been organized. Its linear coaching techniques are easy to follow for beginners. The gradual coordinated breathing characteristics are significantly healing. Athletes and crippled folks alike can practice all or selected exercises to benefit their health, whatever their daily lifestyle requires. Unfolding a Chinese puzzle box reveals its treasures and more Liangong practice reveals more profound comfort.

Doria Cook Nelson
Malibu, CA

I would like to thank you for the exceptional classes I attended at the NWMAF ST '99. Learning and practicing the basics of the Liangong have made a great change in my training. I recently tested for my black stripe in tae kwon do and testing usually makes me a ball of nerves. But this time, I practiced the Liangong over and over prior to the test and then did it mentally until it was my time. I have to say, and my Master Park agreed, this was one of my best tests. By remembering what you told us, I was able to focus on what was inside and was actually able to keep my tension to a minimum.

Lisa Susko
N. Tonawanda, NY

I have found Liangong to be a very useful and effective form of therapeutic exercise both for my patients and myself. Liangong is unique in that it combines the best of Chinese medical theory along with ordinary exercise. Therefore the effects of these exercises are similar to meridian therapy; they simultaneously affect the internal organs' functions as well as all the related muscular and joints and the emotional stresses associated with the meridian. The Liangong exercises are done on positions that align the meridians and allow free flow of the energy through them. The fact that they require no special equipment, and they can be done standing while wearing shoes is a great practical benefit. This means that they can be performed nearly anytime, anywhere. They systematically cover the whole body. Section 1 stretches particular problem areas, while Section 2 seems to integrate the body and pattern the muscles to optimize function.

There is a trend in modern rehabilitation therapy to isolate only the symptomatic areas and treat it separately from the rest of the body. However, this is not how the body works; it functions as a whole with nearly the whole body participating in every motion. To ease movements and improve efficiency, isolated muscle strength is not enough; there needs to be a synergy of muscle function so that the sum of their activity results in increased strength and stamina with less perceived effort. Ordinary exercise therapy does this only haphazardly. Liangong has this integral aspect designed into it from the very beginning.

For special therapeutic use, particular exercises can also be prescribed to aid particular problems. For example, keyboard overuse is nearly a universal problem with my patients. Either they

TESTIMONIALS

have difficulty typing or they strain their finger and wrist using the mouse. These result in shortened pectoral muscles, forward head position, a collapsed upper body posture and flattened carpal tunnels. Exercise 2 of the first series simultaneously corrects all these if repeated periodically during computer work. However, the entire series is so well-balanced that a program of repeating it would be highly recommended.

Liangong has a unique feature: It functions as an "adjustment" to the body. The small contraction at the peak of each exercise, I believe, heightens neurological activity of the body for an instant and allows the nervous system to reprogram itself to maintain a better aligned position. Often after a chiropractic treatment, a patient will feel a little sore or fatigued for a day before feeling better. This is usually a sign of a change in posture and muscle usage that occurs when the body is corrected. I believe Liangong functions as a self-administrated "mini-adjustment." It places the body in a position of correction and change in breathing. The key points are that one can do it in a very safe and comfortable manner.

As a chiropractor myself I can see the inherent genius in the design of the Liangong exercises. Liangong is a perfect supplement to chiropractic care. These exercises enhance the effect of chiropractic treatment and make them longer lasting. The Liangong exercises affect the entire body, correcting individual body parts as well as improving the coordinated function of the body as a unit. They offer therapeutic benefit to muscles, joints, and connective tissue. They improve nerve function by opening the natural pathway for the nerve and relieve impingement. They directly affect the acupuncture meridian system and through it help balance internal organ function and emotional stress.

Personally, Liangong helps me deal with the stress of a very busy chiropractic practice, and busy home life raising two small children. In addition, after 26 years of martial arts practice and numerous injuries incurred along the way, Liangong has helped me improve my physical condition and reduce the effects of previous injury. I thank Master Wen-Mei Yu for teaching me this marvelous health system.

Liangong has gleaned the best of traditional Chinese exercise therapies and combined them with modern scientific exercise theory to form a method I feel is unmatched in the Western world.

Dr. Mark Adachi, D.C.
Glendale, CA

Liangong practice has been a daily part of my life for over two years. The exercises have helped me achieve a sense of well-being despite difficult personal circumstances, although I was not seeking this when I began to learn it. Sometimes my day starts with a sense of sadness or being overwhelmed at my circumstances, but soon after I begin my 20-minute morning practice, that feeling changes. I feel qi begin to flow and I am aware of a sense of well-being.

I am also using counseling, Rolfing, and physical therapy to work my way through these circumstances. Liangong seems to support the healing that each of these approaches promotes; for example, I have a problem with pain and tightness in my neck and shoulders. My Rolfer suggested that I talk to my shoulders and try to learn what I am holding within those tense muscles. My counselor helped me talk through this, so that I could begin to see what situation made me react with tense muscles. Then my Liangong teacher, Debbie Leung, spent an entire Liangong review class on keeping the shoulders relaxed, correct shoulder position, and paying attention to the difference between the tightening and relaxing portions of the exercise. She also accompanied me to a physical therapy appointment, where we worked more on the Liangong exercises specifically for my body.

Liangong helps increase my awareness of the alignment issue that my physical therapist is trying to get me to correct. It supports my Rolfing and physical therapy treatments so I can progress faster. All this work on my body makes me more physically comfortable and centered to work on the mental and emotional discomfort that counseling brings up in me.

Although I am still working on these problems, I feel the relaxation portion of each Liangong exercise has helped me become more aware of the ways I hold tension. I now feel more settled in by body and I am learning to move from my core rather than from the extremities. Of course, this also helps me feel more settled in my mind.

There are a few smaller, more specific benefits as well. I feel less anxious when I am in steep or exposed places — on a roof, or in the mountains — perhaps because Liangong helped me learn where to focus my attention. Recently, I went on a long bike ride with a group of people. On a long steep hill I noticed that other riders were breathing very fast and shallowly, while my breathing was deeper and slower even though I was working just as hard. I think Liangong breathing contributed to this.

Shelley Kirk Rudeen
Olympia, WA

TESTIMONIALS

I began learning Liangong to help my back. My massage therapist said that my back pain was from my sacroiliac joint "getting stuck." It gave me so much pain that it was one of the reasons I retired from farming after almost 20 years. Liangong not only has helped there, it also helped with my bursitis associated with my hip joint, which had been giving me problems for two years. I felt stiff along the side of my leg after sitting and it was tender to the touch. Liangong actually made the bursitis completely go away. I had one day of pain where the bursitis problem was, but after a day of laying off and taking Ibuprofen, it steadily improved. After seven days, I no longer felt any stiffness there. I try to do the exercises two-to-three times a week and more if I am particularly active. I can say that my whole sense of energy and movement has improved.

Betsie DeWreede
Olympia, WA

LIANGONG FOR SPORTS INJURIES

I have practiced Liangong for many years, mostly to maintain health. However, there were times when I used Liangong to help me rehabilitate various sports injuries.

I had chronic problems with my left knee because of torn cartilage and stretched ligaments. One time, after sitting in a kneeling position, I experienced enough pain in the knee to cause me to limp. The next evening, I went to a Liangong workshop and followed the instructions carefully while listening to my body. Even though deep knee bends are not usually recommended for injured knees, I decided to trust the "Bend, Squat, and Stretch Legs" exercise and try to squat completely if my body let me. It did in that exercise as well as the others. After a night's sleep, I was able to walk smoothly with only some residual stiffness.

I was working on a new entrance to a jump during practice at the ice rink where I train as an adult competitive figure skater. After many repetitions, I began to experience pain in my lower back. When I took off my skates at the end of the session, I realized I could barely walk. I had to limp along slowly with my upper body bent forward. At home, I slowly and carefully practiced Liangong to see how it could help me. I found several exercises that seemed to stretch in just the right places. The next day, I could walk normally although there was a lingering stiffness. I could skate if I warmed up with the Liangong exercises that helped the most. From a session with my massage therapist, I learned that the problem was a rotation in my sacroiliac joint, which she was able to fix, removing any lingering stiffness.

Another time, I was working extra hard on improving my cardiovascular strength. For hours afterward, my lungs hurt to breathe. I thought I'd try repeating the last exercise, "Extend Arms and Spread Chest," which was designed to help the lungs. Many hours later, in the evening, I realized that I had completely forgotten about my sore lungs all afternoon, most likely because, shortly after doing the exercise, they no longer hurt.

Debbie Leung
Olympia, WA

SPREAD WINGS TO FLY

I lift my elbows, backward arc.
Shoulders roll like stones
In the surf, up and over, smoother.

Lighter. Rising sharp as wings
Of a tern from the crest
Of an aqua swell, my arms unfurl.

Even a quince branch cut
from the root absorbs the motion
of water. The soul, a blossom

hold the sky, expanding
slower that the eye
can see. This, my life, wild

branch of thorns a hummingbird
shimmers near to drink
from the heart of nectar.

My heart. My wings.

Janet E. Aalfs, Northhampton, Mass.

THE BENEFITS OF LIANGONG PRACTICE
By Janet E. Aalfs

Since 1993, students and teachers of Valley Women's Martial Arts, Inc., a non-profit school and community organization located in western Massachusetts, have been benefiting from the practice of Liangong. Now a branch member of Master Wen-Mei Yu's Jian Mei Internal Martial Arts, VWMA was founded in 1977 and teaches shuri-ryu Okinawan karate, Filipino modern arnis, self-defense, and internal martial arts.

TESTIMONIALS

One black belt instructor of VWMA remembers an injury that was not responding to chiropractic and other treatments. She had fallen down a set of stairs and jammed her shoulder joint, suffering pain for more than a year in her shoulders and neck. Then she began learning Liangong. After six weeks of practicing the first section for the upper body, she was back to full movement and the pain was gone.

Another student has learned over several years of regular practice how to not overextend her joints, thereby avoiding injury. She noticed that the tissue around and inside her relatively loose joints has strengthened and become healthier. Other practitioners have felt improvements such as being able to swing a heavy hammer all day without pain; calming down, moving through anxiety, and feeling empowered by the group's energy; and improved sleep and focusing abilities.

Greater extension, better alignment, increased understanding of movement, and deeper balance through breathing awareness are all benefits that those who do Liangong on a regular basis have experienced. For many people it is especially enjoyable and expansive to practice outdoors. However, these exercises can be done in a variety of spaces such as an office, a train station, airport, or a room at home. And though at 6-feet-1 I didn't really need more height, I'm happy to note that I've lengthened a bit since beginning Liangong. Even more notable is the fact that I no longer get serious stiff necks. Every once in a while I'll have a twinge but it doesn't last. I can feel the self-adjusting action of the movements keeping energy channels clear.

I've been having a great deal of success teaching Liangong to young and old alike, people with a wide range of abilities and disabilities. These exercises are adaptable in any number of ways. For instance, if someone is not able to stand, he may practice sitting or lying down. From one or two exercises to the full sequence, everyone can find some aspect of Liangong that serves to inspire, invigorate, and relax the body, mind, and spirit through mindful movement.

THE FOLLOWING COMMENTS COME FROM MEMBERS OF THE NAPA VALLEY TAI CHI CLUB IN OREGON.

Liangong has increased my flexibility and has helped me to maintain my good health. After exercising, I have a greater feeling of well-being.
— Dixie Paussa

Liangong is a wonderful exercise to build energy and relax.
— Juliane Han

Having severe osteoporosis, I have a relaxed and all-over limber feeling throughout my body after doing Liangong. I know it is making my bones stronger.
— Dorothy Cowger

My joints and balance were very bad — Since doing tai chi and Liangong there has been great improvement and much enjoyment.
— Billie Bingham

I think the Liangong and tai chi have strengthened my knees — the pain in my left knee is gone. My balance has improved. I have a feeling of well-being.
— Barbara Titus

The Liangong exercises give me energy and strength for my fight with cancer. The tai chi gives me strength to move forward with my life.
— Marynell Durbin

Liangong – At age 80 these exercises are very helpful in maintaining mobility without pain.
— Audrey Jones

Having a bad back most of my life, the Liangong exercises for the lower back give much relief.
— Imogene Egner

Liangong and tai chi keep me moving and help my arthritis very much.
— Jesse Bonds

Liangong has helped to eliminate my hip pain and stiffness and strengthened all the muscles used.
— Marcia Suryan

Liangong Joint Rotations – I am 81 years old and these joint rotations keep me flexible in the legs, hips and shoulders. Thank you.
— Lois J. Williams

TESTIMONIALS

The Liangong exercises have helped with my flexibility and balance. — Virginia Huffman

Liangong and tai chi help my body and spirit. — Nobuko Rhodes

Liangong makes me feel better. It is a gentle way to stay flexible and strong. — Jan Hackett

The Liangong Joint Rotations always help my muscle soreness due to hiking, biking, weightlifting or any other activity I am busy with at the time. — Jean Cassinerio

Doing Liangong I feel much younger and healthier. Thank you. — Michiko Chwistek

Liangong has helped me release a lot of tension in my lower back and hence my lower back problems keep getting better. These have helped more than other exercises I had tried previously! — Steve Stefanki

At 90 years of age, Liangong really helps me concentrate. — Christine Roberts

Liangong exercises are especially good for an older person — they are specific to areas that need help, but mild enough for anyone. — Alice Lucas

Tai chi helps my spiritual well-being. I feel good after doing the Liangong exercises. — Pamela Forstner

I am normally a slow-moving person and find that my energy level and feeling of general well-being have increased since taking tai chi. Liangong has helped me with a nervous breathing condition and cuts down leg swelling and leg cramps. The whole experience has been tremendously positive. — Lucy Moris

I had bronchitis for years and I started doing Liangong and the Wild Goose Chi Gung and breathing from the stomach up through the chest. I have not had the bronchitis since. — Martha Dowd

I often come to class at 10 a.m. after working a 12-hour night shift as an R.N. Tai chi and Liangong are fantastic ways to revitalize and/or relax. Wonderful. — Bob Adams

At age 65, my body responds to Liangong practice by improving my flexibility and giving me a sense of calmness and well-being. It gets to those parts of my body that are usually neglected. I also meet a lot of great people. — Pete Capovilla

Liangong exercises are strength builders and have been helpful to me. I am a 69-year-old woman who has been bothered by a weak lower back. Since I began tai chi and Liangong practice three years ago, my body is stronger, my mind is calmer and my back is much improved. — Joan A. Bartlett

My blood pressure, which was elevated, is normal now since doing tai chi and Liangong. — Betty Forstner

Tai chi and Liangong have made my whole body and mind feel so much better, relaxed, stronger; and my attitude about life is greater. While I cannot remember some of the movements, I can follow and feel any movement is good for me. Another thing: the people in the class are so warm and friendly. Thank you. — Gladys Langdon

Liangong helps me to relax and prepare for the tai chi that follows. — Kitty Kersten

I always feel noticeably more fluid after the Liangong exercises. They loosen the tight muscles and joints. I also find they are easily done as I go about my chores indoors and out. They are very beneficial to my well-being. — Rosemary Gallager

Liangong helps aid movement in my knee and hip joints. I used them to help prepare for my black belt test! — Joellen Hiltbrand

Liangong gives me a sense of breath and connection to my body. — Andrea Weber

Liangong and tai chi keep me from going completely bonkers! — Dana Price

ABOUT THE AUTHOR
— WEN-MEI YU

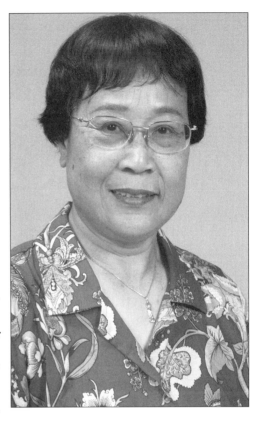

Born in Shanghai, China, in 1936, Wen-Mei Yu was diagnosed with a bleeding ulcer at age 17. At the time, both Eastern and Western medicine were ineffective. Her family and friends urged her to try chi kung (qigong). Although reluctant, she tried to follow basic, simple methods of chi kung practice. In a very short time, she had great improvement in her health. This led to a personal journey of self-discovery, where she dedicated her life to the study of internal arts, such as taijiquan, chi kung and related internal arts systems.

Wen-Mei Yu learned Wild Goose (or Dayan) Chi Kung directly from Yang Mei Jun, a modern-day exponent of the Taoist Kunlun School. Along with Wild Goose Chi Kung, she studied several forms and systems of chi kung, including contemporary forms such as Guo Ling Chi Kung with Guo Ling and Soaring Crane Chi Kung with Zhao Jin Xiang. Traditional systems of study included Wei Tuo Chi Kung (Buddhist Shaolin) and Wild Goose Chi Kung. Wen-Mei Yu also had the privilege of studying in great detail the Liangong health exercise system developed by Dr. Zhuang Yuan Ming.

Recipient of the All China Excellent Wushu Coach Award in 1983, Wen-Mei Yu is also highly noted for her practice of taijiquan (tai chi chuan). She studied the Wu style of taijiquan and weapons with Wu Jian Quan's eldest daughter, Wu Ying Huan, and Wu Jian Quan's son-in-law, Ma Yueh Liang. She studied Yang style taijiquan and weapons with Fu Zhong Wen (a student of the legendary Chen

Fake), whose books and materials on the subject of taijiquan continue to enlighten people to this day. She also studied Chen style taijiquan and contemporary forms of taijiquan with Zhou Yuan Long, whose drawings of Chen Fake, Chen Zhaokwei, Yang Cheng Fu, Hao Shao Ru, Jiang Rong Qiao, Wu Jian Quan, and the 24 simplified version of taijiquan (to name a few) continue to be used for a variety of books, periodicals and publications. Wen-Mei Yu is a Wu style taijiquan stylist, a senior member of the Chian Chuan Tai Chi Chuan Association, and has been a recognized active member and student since 1974.

Wen-Mei Yu came to the United States in 1987 at the invitation of the International Kung Fu Federation. Not one to sit on her laurels, Wen-Mei Yu competed and won first place in Hand Forms at the 2nd American Tai Chi Championships in San Francisco in 1989 and first place in Taiji Hands and Taiji Weapons Forms competitions at the World Cup in Los Angeles in 1989.

She is the recipient of the "Award of Excellence" from the National Women's Martial Arts Federation. Internationally, she has served as an instructor at the Women's Martial Arts Festival of Canada and for the Feminist International Summer Training Festival (also known as F.I.S.T.) held in the Netherlands and Europe. She has lectured and taught private lessons, group classes, and seminars throughout the world. She has taught people from various walks of life and abilities, including medical and health professionals; accident victims; cancer patients; people with special needs (including disabilities); and others seeking personal development and enlightenment.

Wen-Mei Yu regularly returns to China to continue her studies in taijiquan, chi kung and related internal arts to delve deeper into the tradition, as well as to keep up on contemporary research and developments in her chosen styles. She was recognized as "Writer of the Year" by *Inside Kung-Fu* magazine in 1994 and named "Woman of the Year" by the same publication in 1997.